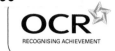
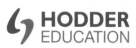

Official Publisher Partnership

HOME ECONOMICS
OCR FOOD AND NUTRITION FOR GCSE

Anita Tull

Consultants: Lyndsey Jackson and Jan Shally

HODDER
EDUCATION
AN HACHETTE UK COMPANY

Orders: please contact Bookpoint Ltd, 130 Milton Park, Abingdon, Oxon OX14 4SB. Telephone: (44) 01235 827720. Fax: (44) 01235 400454. Lines are open from 9.00 – 5.00, Monday to Saturday, with a 24-hour message answering service. You can also order through our website www.hoddereducation.co.uk

If you have any comments to make about this, or any of our other titles, please send them to educationenquiries@hodder.co.uk

British Library Cataloguing in Publication Data
A catalogue record for this title is available from the British Library

ISBN: 978 0 340 98397 3

First Edition Published 2009
This Edition Published 2010
Impression number   10 9 8 7 6 5 4
Year   2012 2011 2010

Copyright © 2009 Anita Tull

Hachette UK's policy is to use papers that are natural, renewable and recyclable products and made from wood grown in sustainable forests. The logging and manufacturing processes are expected to conform to the environmental regulations of the country of origin.

Cover photo © Simon Marcus/Corbis.
Typeset by Pantek Arts Ltd., Maidstone, Kent.
Illustrations by Oxford Designers and Illustrators
Printed in Italy for Hodder Education, an Hachette UK Company, 338 Euston Road, London NW1 3BH

CONTENTS

ABOUT THIS BOOK

This book has been written specifically for the OCR GCSE Home Economics (Food and Nutrition) course. The content has been organised to match the qualification specification, to help guide you through the requirements of the course.

The course is divided into three parts, and the book is set out in the same way:
- Unit B001: Food and Nutrition Short Tasks
- Unit B002: Food Study Tasks
- Unit B003: Principles of Food and Nutrition.

Unit B001: Food and Nutrition Short tasks will guide you through the process of planning, carrying out, recording and evaluating a Short Task. The book works through each stage of the process using two realistic Short Task examples (a Practical Task and an Investigative Task) as guides.

Unit B002: Food Study Tasks is divided into three topics (Research; Planning and carrying out practical tasks; Evaluation and drawing conclusions) which guide you through the process, again using a realistic example as a guide.

Unit B003: Principles of Food and Nutrition contains all the underpinning knowledge you will need to help you understand the subject so you can prepare for your written exam and be able to apply theory to practice in both the Short Tasks and the Food Study Task.

To help you ensure that all topics have been covered, Unit B003 is divided into seven parts, with individual topics within each part:
- Nutrition and health
- Food commodities
- Meal planning
- Food preparation and cooking
- Food safety and preservation
- Consumer education.

These are set out in manageable sections to help you work steadily and systematically through the information. In addition, there is a section on Preparing for a written exam.

The main aim has been to produce a source of information that is detailed but easy to use. The topics are explained clearly and you are provided with lots of opportunities to test your knowledge and understanding as you work through the course. There are lots of interesting activities included to help assess your learning as well as practice for examination assessments.

We hope you enjoy your course and learn lots about food and nutrition. Good luck!

 Teachers: where you see this icon, additional exercises are available at www.hodderplus.co.uk/foodandnutrition. Answers to activities are also available there.

ACKNOWLEDGEMENTS

Every effort has been made to trace the copyright holders of material reproduced here. The authors and publishers would like to thank the following for permission to reproduce copyright illustrations:

P.2 Chris Hondros/Getty Images; p.5 BEN STANSALL/AFP/Getty Images; p.15 (bottom) Nutrition Systems www.compeat.co.uk; p.19 Andrew Callaghan/Hodder Education; p.20 (top) Martyn F. Chillmaid, (bottom) Andrew Callaghan/Hodder Education; p.21 © Courtney Keating/iStockphoto.com; p.31 © George Bailey/iStockphoto.com; p.33 (top) © Liv Friis-Larsen/iStockphoto.com, (bottom) © Dan Bachman/iStockphoto.com; p.38 (left) ©Morgan Lane Photography/iStockphoto.com, (right) studiomode/Alamy; p.39 © iStockphoto.com; p.40 (top) © Photolibrary.Com, (bottom) © Donald Erickson/iStockphoto.com; p.41 © Linda & Colin McKie/iStockphoto.com; p.42 (top) Maximilian Stock Ltd/Photolibrary.com, (bottom) © Stockbyte/Getty Images; p.44 © Daniel Loiselle/iStockphoto.com; p.48 © techno/iStockphoto.com; p.51 DR M.A. ANSARY/SCIENCE PHOTO LIBRARY; p.52 SCIENCE PHOTO LIBRARY; p.53 Emotive Images/Photolibrary.com; p.54 © Elena Elisseeva/iStockphoto.com; p.55 BIOPHOTO ASSOCIATES/SCIENCE PHOTO LIBRARY; p.56 DEA/G.CIGOLINI/Getty Images; p.58 (top) © www.j-photo.co.uk/iStockphoto.com, (bottom) WESTMINSTER HOSPITAL/SCIENCE PHOTO LIBRARY; p.61 (top) Chris Pancewicz/Alamy; p.62 © Ivan Mateev/iStockphoto.com; p.63 Neil Fletcher and Matthew Ward/Dorling Kindersley/Getty Images; p.67 Food Standards Agency; p.68 (top) © Stockbyte/Getty Images, (middle) © Photodisc/Getty Images, (bottom) Philip Wilkins/Photolibrary.com; p.72 © Ana Abejon/iStockphoto.com; p.84 Food Standards Agency; p.94 (top) © Sascha Burkard/iStockphoto.com, (middle) © Jacek Chabraszewski/iStockphoto.com; p.95 (top) © Aldo Murillo/iStockphoto.com, (bottom) © Eliza Snow/iStockphoto.com; p.96 © Mikhail Kokhanchikov/iStockphoto.com; pp.100–1 Sam Bailey/Hodder Education; p.102 (top) Stockbyte/Photolibrary Group Ltd, (middle) © Iain Sarjeant/iStockphoto.com; p.103 Damir Begovic/StockFood Creative/Getty Images; p.104 ICP/Alamy; fig. 107 Martyn F. Chillmaid; p.114 © Photodisc/Getty Images, © Ingram Publishing Limited; p.116 (top) © Daniel Tero/iStockphoto.com, (bottom) © Long Tran The/iStockphoto.com; p.117 (top) © Thomas Perkins/iStockphoto.com; p.119 © Claudio Baldini/iStockphoto.com; p.120 (top) © Mona Makela/iStockphoto.com, (bottom) © arteretum, www.joannawnuk.com/iStockphoto.com; p.125 (bottom) ISSOUF SANOGO/AFP/Getty Images; p.130 Food Standards Agency; p.133 © Photodisc/Getty Images; p.134 © yong hong - Fotolia.com; p.135 imagebroker/Alamy; p.136 ACE STOCK LIMITED/Alamy; p.138 www.purestockX.com; p.140 (top) Image Source Black/Alamy; p.142 (top) © Ethan Myerson/iStockphoto.com, (bottom) © Catherine Yeulet/iStockphoto.com; p.145 © Ed Hidden/iStockphoto.com; p.146 © Alexander Hafemann/iStockphoto.com; p.147 (top) ShaunFinch/Alamy, (middle) The Vegetarian Society, (bottom) © Vikram Raghuvanshi/iStockphoto.com; p.148 Andrew Callaghan/Hodder Education; p.149 (top) ©Photodisc/Getty Images, (bottom) MARK SYKES/SCIENCE PHOTO LIBRARY; p.150 Andrew Callaghan/Hodder Education; p.151 Stephen Barnes Food and Drink/Alamy; p.153 (top) © Dave White/iStockphoto.com, (bottom) Andy Crawford/Dorling Kindersley/Getty Images; p.154 (top) DR P. MARAZZI/SCIENCE PHOTO LIBRARY, (bottom) © Photodisc/Getty Images; p.155 © Stockbyte/Getty Images; p.170 © Jason Lugo/iStockphoto.com; p.171 (top) Sarah Bailey/Hodder Education, (bottom) Shimon & Tammar/Photolibrary.com; p.172 © Ingram Publishing Limited; p.175 (top left) Dorling Kindersley/Getty Images, (bottom left) Neil Holmes Freelance Digital/Alamy, (middle) Daily Grind/Alamy, (right) Tefal; p.176 © George Peters/iStockphoto.com; p.179 (top) Sarah Bailey/Hodder Education, (bottom) Andrew Callaghan/Hodder Education; p.182 (top) Sarah Bailey/Hodder Education, (bottom) Sam Bailey/Hodder Education; pp.183–5 Sarah Bailey/Hodder Education; p.186 (top) © Photodisc/Getty Images, (others) © Image Source/Getty Images; p.187 (top) © Stockbyte/Getty Images, (others) © Image Source/Getty Images; p.188 (top) Phil Degginger/Alamy, (others) Anthony Blake/Photolibrary.com; p.189 (top) © MARIA TOUTOUDAKI/iStockphoto.com, (bottom) Sarah Bailey/Hodder Education; p.191 Andrew Callaghan/Hodder Education; p.192 (top two) Sam Bailey/Hodder Education, (third) Andrew Callaghan/Hodder Education, (bottom) Jerry Young/Dorling Kindersley/Getty Images; p.193 (top) © Owen Price/iStockphoto.com, (middle) © Ingram Publishing Limited, (bottom) Sam Bailey/Hodder Education; p.194 Andrew Callaghan/Hodder Education; p.197 Sarah Bailey/Hodder Education; p.206 Adel A. Kader, Department of Plant Sciences, MS2, University of California; p.207 SCIMAT/SCIENCE PHOTO LIBRARY; p.208 (bottom) EYE OF SCIENCE/SCIENCE PHOTO LIBRARY; p.210 (middle) © Miroslaw Modzelewski/iStockphoto.com; p.219 Bananastock/Photolibrary Group Ltd; p.224 (top) © Photodisc/Getty Images, (bottom) © The Image Works/TopFoto; p.227 Helene Rogers/Alamy; p.228 Food Standards Agency; p.229 (Red Tractor) Assured Food Standards, (Freedom Food) RSPCA; p.230 shaun d parrin/photographersdirect.com.

Crown copyright material is reproduced with the permission of the Controller of HMSO and the Queen's Printer for Scotland. Dietary reference values are taken from COMA, 'Dietary Reference Values for Food Energy and Nutrients for the United Kingdom' (Department of Health, 1991).

INTRODUCTION

During your GCSE Food and Nutrition course you will be expected to complete three short tasks. Two of the tasks will be practical tasks and the other one will be an investigative task (these are explained later in this section on page 2). Both types of task involve practical work.

You will be given a set of task titles to choose from and your teacher will help you choose the most suitable ones for you.

The aim of the short tasks is to enable you to apply, in a practical situation, the knowledge you have gained in your lessons, as the chart below explains.

Sections of the short tasks that your teacher will assess	Which knowledge and practical skills the short tasks will test you on.
Planning the task	• The choices of practical work and recipes you make • Your reasons for choosing your practical work • Your skill at writing a timed plan of practical work • The methods you use for recording the results of your practical work
Practical work	• How well you follow your timed plan of work and make use of the time available • How well and effectively you organise your work space, equipment and ingredients • How cleanly and tidily you work and your attention to food hygiene • How safely and independently you use kitchen equipment • How many different cooking methods you use and how well you use them • How many types of skills you demonstrate, including practical cookery skills, ICT skills, costing and taste testing
Outcomes of the practical work	• The quality of the practical work you make and how well you present it • How well you carry out some tasting panels for your practical work and how accurately you record the results
Evaluation of the task	• Your ability to identify the strengths and weaknesses of all aspects of your completed short task • Your ability to suggest how you could improve the work, with reasons • What conclusions you have drawn from the short task

On the following pages, each part of the short tasks is explained and examples are used to guide you through the process and help you to achieve the best result you can.

TYPES OF SHORT TASKS

Practical tasks

These tasks specify (tell you) what practical work to prepare, e.g:

- Plan and make two food items.
- Plan and make a meal.
- Plan and make some items for a packed lunch box.
- Plan and make one sweet and one savoury dish.

These will be related to a particular theme. Here are some examples:

- the importance of particular nutrients
- following dietary guidelines
- providing food for particular age groups
- providing food for particular health conditions
- using specific food commodities such as fish, meat or eggs
- providing food for particular religious or cultural differences
- demonstrating cake-making methods
- using a specific piece of kitchen equipment
- the importance of food hygiene when preparing food.

Investigative tasks

These tasks give you a general theme (like the ones above) and ask you to investigate it and plan your own practical work to illustrate it. You are also required to plan and carry out suitable methods of testing, assessing and recording the results of your investigation and practical work:

- nutritional analysis using a computer program
- taste testing panels
- surveys
- costing
- sensory testing.

Here are examples of a practical task title and an investigative task title.

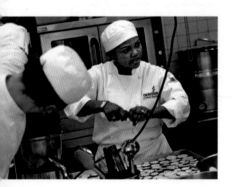

Practical task:	**Investigative task:**
Protein is an important nutrient for the growth, repair and maintenance of the body. Plan and cook two dishes that would provide protein for a person who follows a vegetarian diet. Support your choices with nutritional data. Evaluate your work.	Plan and carry out an investigation into the advantages and disadvantages of using ready-made food products compared to homemade products that use fresh ingredients. Record and display your results, using them as evidence on which to base your conclusions. Evaluate your work.

In the following pages these two examples are used to explain how to carry out the short tasks, so that you understand what to do.

Here are a few general tips and guidelines to help you:

Get started! – The most successful students are the ones who start work straightaway when they have been given their task. Read through the task carefully and highlight the key words. Make some notes or lists on what you need to do. Keep these notes in a safe place so you can keep referring to them.

Be organised! – The most successful students are the ones who keep their written work in a file, in a logical order and plan their practical work in advance so that they have all the materials they need. They then hand work in to their teachers for ongoing assessment. They also know where to find out information.

Working on your own – The work that you present for each task must be your own and not copied from anywhere or anyone else. If you are struggling for ideas or information, ask for help from your teacher.

Practise your practical work – This will make you feel confident about presenting your work for each short task, knowing that you are able to produce good results.

Evaluate as you go along – Think about how you do your planning, any problems you have and how you overcome them. Keep a note so that you can use this in your evaluation. Also, think about how you do your practical work, any changes you make to your timed plan and make a note for your evaluation.

PLANNING YOUR SHORT TASK

UNDERSTANDING AND INTERPRETING THE TASK

The first job to do when you are given your task is to read it carefully and highlight the key words, as shown below for our two examples.

Practical task

Protein is an important nutrient for the growth, repair and maintenance of the body.

Plan and cook two main course dishes that would provide protein for a person who follows a vegetarian diet.

Support your choices with nutritional data.

Evaluate your work.

Investigative task

Plan and carry out an investigation into the advantages and disadvantages of using ready-made food products compared to homemade products that use fresh ingredients. Record and display your results, using them as evidence on which to base your conclusions.

Evaluate your work.

Highlighting key words helps to focus your attention on what you need to do.

Make sure that you refer back to the original question at regular intervals to check that you are doing what it asks you to do. It is easy to get sidetracked and do something that you were not asked to do (or forget something that you were asked to do).

The second job is to look at the highlighted words and make notes about what you understand them to mean and how you are going to interpret (explain what you are going to do) the task. The diagram below shows the sort of notes you would make.

The dishes need to be based on animal protein foods (cheese, eggs, milk), and plant protein foods (peas, beans, lentils)

Should be savoury, contain plenty of protein and be filling

Say how the chosen dishes have provided enough protein for a vegetarian – use the nutritional data to support this. If possible ask some vegetarians to try the dishes and evaluate them for flavour, colour, texture and so on. Say if the dishes or the task could have been improved

Practical task

Protein is an important nutrient for the growth, repair and maintenance of the body.

Plan and cook two main course dishes that would provide protein for a person who follows a vegetarian diet.

Support your choices with nutritional data.

Evaluate your work.

Ovo-lacto vegetarians eat animal products such as dairy foods

Use a nutrient analyser programme to analyse how much protein is in the dishes and compare this to the dietary reference values (DRVs) for adults and children

Time, cost, convenience, ingredients used, nutritional value

Compare time taken to make food to time saved during the week when ready meals are used

Meals should be substantial for all the family and should provide a variety of nutrients

Investigative task

Plan and carry out an investigation into the advantages and disadvantages of using ready-made food products compared to homemade products that use fresh ingredients. Record and display your results, using them as evidence on which to base your conclusions.

Evaluate your work.

Cook chill, frozen, takeaway

Set up a tasting panel

CHOOSING AND CARRYING OUT SUITABLE PRACTICAL WORK

Your third job is to decide what practical work you will carry out. You will need to take into account the following things when choosing your practical work:

- the amount of time you have available to prepare and cook the dishes
- the amount of money you are going to spend on the ingredients
- the availability of ingredients
- the equipment and space you have available to work with
- the number of skills you are going to demonstrate
- the way you will present your work
- the way you will carry out any tasting panels.

It is a good idea to make a list of possible dishes and to show these to your teacher who can help you to select the most suitable ones.

Suggestions for the practical task

Here are some suggestions for our two example tasks.

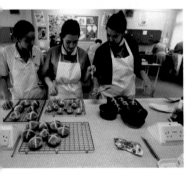

Practical task

Protein is an important nutrient for the growth, repair and maintenance of the body.

Plan and cook two dishes that would provide protein for a person who follows a vegetarian diet. Support your choices with nutritional data.

Evaluate your work.

Suggested main course dishes:

- pasta with cheese sauce
- vegetable lasagne
- tomato and cheese pizza
- vegetable curry with chickpeas
- lentil dhal.

Here are the chosen recipes (each of them serves four people).

Pasta with cheese sauce

Ingredients:
200g penne pasta
1 tbsp vegetable oil
1 clove garlic, crushed
1 small leek, thinly sliced
150g button mushrooms, thinly sliced
100g frozen peas, thawed

Cheese sauce:
50g butter
50g plain flour
500mls whole milk
150g grated mature cheddar cheese

You need a square or round heatproof dish to bake this in.

Method:

1. Boil pasta in large pan of water until tender. Drain off the water.

2. Heat oil in frying pan and cook garlic, leeks and mushrooms until leek softens.

3. Mix pasta and leek mixture together in a bowl with the peas.

4. Sauce: melt butter in a pan and stir in flour. Cook for 1 minute and remove from heat. Add the milk gradually and return to heat, stirring all the time until boiled and thickened. Remove from heat and stir in the cheese until melted.

5. Stir a third of the sauce into the vegetable mixture and place it into a large ovenproof dish.

6. Pour remaining sauce over the top and place under hot grill until golden brown.

Lentil dhal

Ingredients:
50g ghee or oil
1 clove garlic, crushed
½ tsp finely chopped fresh chilli
½ tsp finely chopped root ginger
1 tsp powdered turmeric
1 tsp garam masala
½ tsp salt
1 tsp ground coriander
1 tbsp fresh coriander leaves, finely chopped
1 star anise
1 small cinnamon stick
1 tsp mustard
1 tomato, chopped finely
1 medium onion, chopped finely
1 stick celery, chopped finely
1 litre water
500g orange lentils

Method:

1. Heat the ghee or oil in a large, heavy-based saucepan.

2. Add the garlic, chilli and ginger, all the spices and herbs, mustard, tomato, onion and celery.

3. Fry for about 10 minutes until well blended.

4. Add the water and bring to the boil.

5. Stir the lentils in and cook on a low heat for about half an hour, until the lentils are soft, stirring occasionally.

6. If the dhal becomes too thick before the lentils are soft, add some more water.

Suggestions for investigative task

Investigative task

Plan and carry out an investigation into the advantages and disadvantages of using ready-made food products compared to homemade products that use fresh ingredients. Record and display your results, using them as evidence on which to base your conclusions.

Evaluate your work.

Suggested ready-made food products that could be compared with homemade versions (you could choose one or two depending on how much time you have to complete the task):

- cottage pie
- curry
- soups
- lasagne
- savoury flans (quiche)

- pasties
- pies (sweet or savoury)
- cheesecake
- cakes.

When collecting ideas, read through the recipes carefully to make sure that you will have the time and skills to prepare them.

Justifying your choice

The fourth job is to justify your choice of practical work (see below).

Making a timed plan

The fifth job is to make a timed plan for carrying out your practical work (see page 9).

Making your dishes

The sixth job is to carry out your practical work and present the dishes. Here is a reminder of what your teacher will assess you on when you are cooking:

- How well you follow your timed plan of work and make use of the time available.
- How well and effectively you organise your work space, equipment and ingredients.
- How cleanly and tidily you work and your attention to food hygiene.
- How safely and independently you use kitchen equipment.
- How many different cooking methods you use and how well you use them (boiling, steaming, stewing, braising, grilling, baking, frying, microwaving).
- How many types of practical cookery skills you demonstrate. These include skills such as pastry and sauce making, knife skills to prepare fish, meat, fruit or vegetables, bread, scone and cake making.

JUSTIFYING YOUR CHOICE OF PRACTICAL WORK

When you have chosen your practical work, you will need to justify your choices. This means writing down how and why your practical work is suitable for the requirements of the short task you are doing and the reasons you chose them.

The choices for our two examples are justified on the next page.

Practical task

Protein is an important nutrient for the growth, repair and maintenance of the body.

Plan and cook two dishes that would provide protein for a person who follows a vegetarian diet. Support your choices with nutritional data.

Evaluate your work.

Chosen practical work:

- pasta with cheese sauce
- lentil dhal.

The reasons for this choice are as follows.

Pasta with cheese sauce	Lentil dhal
• The dish contains milk and cheese which are good sources of HBV protein. • The vegetables include peas which also contain LBV protein as they are seeds. • The dish is colourful because of the vegetables, and has a variety of flavours due to the vegetables and cheese. • The dish contains a variety of textures from the tender vegetables, the smooth sauce and soft pasta, • The dish is filling and therefore suitable as a main course for vegetarian children or adults. • The chosen dish meets the requirements of the task.	• The lentils and beans provide a good source of LBV protein. • The cheese and milk provide a good source of HBV protein. • The dish has a variety of textures from the vegetables. • The dish is filling and therefore suitable as a main course for vegetarian children or adults. • The chosen dish meets the requirements of the task.

Investigative task

Plan and carry out an investigation into the advantages and disadvantages of using ready-made food products compared to homemade products that use fresh ingredients. Record and display your results, using them as evidence on which to base your conclusions.

Evaluate your work.

Chosen practical work:
• Homemade beef cottage pie – compared in price, preparation time and sensory qualities to a range (cheapest to most expensive) of cook-chill and frozen ready-made beef cottage pies from a range of supermarkets.
• Vegetable soup – compared in price, preparation time and sensory qualities to a range (cheapest to most expensive) of fresh cook-chill, canned, dried and instant soups from a range of supermarkets.

Homemade beef cottage pie	Vegetable soup
• Cottage pie is a familiar and traditional main course dish which is quite easy to make at home using either raw minced beef or leftover meat from a roasted joint of beef. • The cottage pie can be made relatively quickly. • There are several ready-made versions to compare homemade with. • The chosen dish meets the requirements of the task.	• Vegetable soup is a familiar traditional soup which is easy to make at home using a variety of vegetables. • The soup can be made relatively quickly. • There are several ready-made versions to compare homemade with. • The chosen dish meets the requirements of the task.

TOPIC 2

PLANNING AND CARRYING OUT PRACTICAL WORK

A written timed plan of practical work is a good way of demonstrating that you are able to prepare food in a logical order, making the best use of the time available.

It also helps you to remember important things such as oven temperatures and baking times.

In order to write a timed plan of work, you need to:

- Read through your recipes carefully, making note of important points such as oven temperatures, cooking, setting, chilling times and serving information.
- Work out the order in which you need to carry out the processes.
- Include time for clearing up.
- Give realistic times for preparation of ingredients (how long does it take you to peel ten potatoes?).

A timed plan is given for **one** of the example short tasks below.

Practical task

Protein is an important nutrient for the growth, repair and maintenance of the body.

Plan and cook two dishes that would provide protein for a person who follows a vegetarian diet. Support your choices with nutritional data.

Evaluate your work.

Sample timed plan – time allowed to complete practical work – 50 minutes (09.30–10.20). Your teacher may suggest doing two time plans so that you can make each dish in a different session.

Chosen practical work: Pasta with cheese sauce and lentil dhal.

The first column should **describe** what practical activities you will **be doing and the sequence** (order) in which you will be doing them. Use the 'method' section of your recipes to help you write it. In this example, the Pasta with cheese sauce activities are printed in orange and the Dhal activities are printed in blue so that you can see how they have been fitted together into the timed plan.

The second column is to remind you of things you must remember to do and to help you make the recipe successfully.

Time	Activity	Special points
09.30	Peel and chop garlic, leeks and mushrooms	Chop the vegetables into small pieces so that they do not take long to cook
	Peel and finely chop the onion, tomato, celery, ginger and garlic	Light oven – gas 6/200°C
09.39	Boil pasta in large pan of water until tender	Stir the pasta occasionally to stop it sticking together
	Heat the ghee or oil in a large heavy-based saucepan and add the garlic, chilli and ginger, all the spices and herbs, mustard, tomato, onion and celery	
09.42	Fry for about 10 minutes until well blended.	
09.44	Heat oil in frying pan – cook garlic, leeks and mushrooms until leek softens	
09.46	Make sauce: melt butter in a pan and stir in flour and cook for 1 minute and remove from heat	Stir well occasionally to cook evenly
09.47 09.48	Add the milk gradually and return to heat, stirring all the time until boiled and thickened	Stir thoroughly to avoid lumps in the sauce
09.53	Remove from heat and stir in the cheese until melted	Check the flavour of the sauce. Keep the sauce warm with a lid on the pan to prevent a skin from forming.
09.55	Add the boiling water and bring back to the boil	
10.00	Stir the lentils in and cook on a low heat for about half an hour, until the lentils are soft, stirring occasionally	If the dhal becomes too thick before the lentils are soft, add some more water.
10.05	Clear work surface and wash up	
10.08	Check pasta and drain off water	
10.09	Turn off vegetables and mix with peas and pasta in a bowl	
10.12	Stir a third of the sauce into the vegetable mixture and place it into a large ovenproof dish	Wipe the edges of the dish first so that any sauce that has gone on to it does not burn
10.14	Pour remaining sauce over the top and place under hot grill until golden brown	
	Begin final washing up and clearing away	
	Carry on with clearing up	
	Garnish and serve both dishes	

ORGANISING YOUR RESOURCES EFFECTIVELY

In a practical cooking situation, when you have a limited amount of time in which to prepare food, it is important to be well organised.

Good organisation enables you to:

- know where everything is so you do not waste time looking for things
- be focused and clear about what you are doing.

The key points for effective organisation of resources are:

- Collect all your ingredients and equipment together at your work station before you start.

- Clear as you go – wash up regularly, throw rubbish away and wipe the work surface regularly.

- Place ingredients on a tray – put perishable foods in the refrigerator.
- Organise your equipment so that it is easy and safe to use.

USING EQUIPMENT SAFELY, EFFECTIVELY AND INDEPENDENTLY

Kitchen equipment is designed to help make the process of preparing and cooking food easier and more effective. It is important to familiarise yourself with the range of equipment that is available in the kitchen that you work in.

Safety

You must follow basic safety and hygiene rules:

- Chop food on a chopping board and NEVER into your hand.
- Keep knives sharp. Blunt knives are very dangerous.
- Always follow the manufacturer's instructions when using a piece of equipment.
- do not handle electrical equipment with wet hands or use it near water.
- ALWAYS use oven gloves to remove hot items from ovens. NEVER use a wet tea towel or dishcloth as the fabric is too thin and the water will immediately turn to steam and scald you.
- NEVER put your hand or a piece of equipment such as a spoon into a food processor, blender or electric mixer when it is running.
- If a piece of equipment has a guard, make sure it is in place before you use the equipment.
- Keep electrical leads away from a heat source or sharp knives.
- Tie back long hair.

ACTIVITY

Many pieces of equipment have built-in safety features. Look at a food processor and identify the safety features it has.

Food safety

Store perishable foods, such as cream, poultry, fish and meat, in the refrigerator.

If you have them, use the correct coloured chopping board for the right foods.

ACTIVITY

Find out which foods would be prepared on each of these chopping boards.

Red

Yellow

Green

Brown

Blue

White

COSTING YOUR PRACTICAL WORK

In a short task you may need to work out the cost of a food product you have made, and then work out how much a portion or serving costs for one person.

To work this out, this is what you should do (using a chart or grid):

1 Write out the ingredients used in the first column.
2 Write out the total amount of each ingredient used in the second column.
3 Find out the cost of a kilogram or litre of each ingredient (this information is usually displayed on a food label, a price label in a market or a ticket on a supermarket shelf).
4 Work out how much your ingredient costs in the following way, using cheddar cheese as an example:
   • Cheddar cheese costs £7.50 for 1 kilogram
   • 100g of cheese costs £7.50 ÷ 10 = 75p (because there are 10 x 100g in a kilogram)
   • Amount of cheddar cheese used in recipe = 200g
   • Cost of cheese = 75p x 2 = £1.50
5 Once you have worked out all the ingredient prices, add them up to find the total cost of the recipe.
6 Divide the total cost by the number of portions the recipe makes to find the cost of one portion. For example, the total cost for four portions = £10.60. One portion = £10.60 ÷ 4 = £2.65

ACTIVITY

Using the instructions here, work out the total cost of a recipe of your choice, and the cost of one portion.

CARRYING OUT TASTE TESTING

For your short task assessments, you will be required to carry out some taste testing of the food you have made. The results of these tests will help you to write up your evaluation of the short task.

For your short task assessments, you will be required to carry out some taste testing of the food you have made. The results of these tests will help you to write up your evaluation of the short task.

Taste testing of food is a method called sensory analysis which is used to find out:
• whether a food product is acceptable or not
• whether an improvement can be made to a food product
• how long the shelf-life of a food product is.

During the testing, tasters sample some food and then do one or more of the following tests:
• describe it (colour, texture, flavour, smell or what they feel about it)
• rate it (too salty, not sweet enough)
• compare it to another food (which food is crispier or smoother?)
• rank it along with other food products (the most liked and the least liked).

There are a number of tests that can be carried out, some of which are described below. You could use them for your short tasks.

Rating test
What you have to do:

1 Ask some people to volunteer to taste your food product and rate it according to what you want to know – if they like it or how sweet, crisp or chewy it is.
2 Ask them to rate it on a scale as in the examples opposite.

Preference rating (this could be used for either of the short task examples)

Please indicate, by ticking a box below, how much you liked the food product.

I liked it very much	I liked it a little bit	I didn't like or dislike it	I didn't like it much	I didn't like it at all

Order of preference (this could be used for the investigative task example, testing ready-made and homemade food products)

Please indicate by writing the name of each food sample in a box below, according to how you rate them.

1 (the best)	2	3	4	5 (the worst)

The results of your ratings tests could be presented in the form of:

- a table of results
- as percentages ('88 per cent of the testers rated the homemade soup as the best and 9 per cent rated the instant dried soup as the worst')
- a pie chart
- a graph.

Profiling test

This test could be used to find out what people particularly like about your food product, to help you build up a profile of it according to a range of sensory qualities.

What you have to do:

1 Make your food product and ask people to try it.
2 Ask them to give the food product a series of scores out of five (where one is the least/worst and five is the most/best) for a range of sensory qualities, such as: saltiness, smoothness, crispiness, tenderness and lemony flavour.
3 Add up their scores out of five for each quality, and divide that number by the number of people who tried it. This will give you an average score.
4 Present the results on a table, as in the example below.
5 Plot the average scores on a radar graph (you can do this on the computer using the Excel program).
6 Evaluate the product according to the radar graph (see below).

Example: Using our example from the practical task (pasta in cheese sauce), the table below shows how to present the scores for various sensory qualities.

Sensory quality	Tester ratings (out of 5)	Average score
Cheesiness of sauce	4,4,3,5,5,4,4,5,3,5	4.2
Smoothness of sauce	2,2,2,3,3,2,1,4,3,2	2.4
Overall strength of vegetable flavour	1,1,1,2,1,2,2,1,1,1	1.3
Tenderness of vegetables	4,4,4,4,4,5,5,5,3,4	4.2
Attractiveness of colour of finished dish	4,3,3,3,3,5,5,4,5,4	4.1

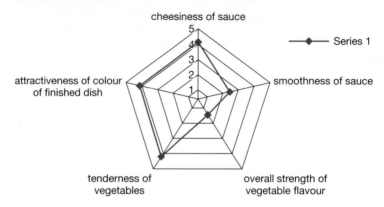

Profile of pasta in cheese sauce

Once you have the profile data, you should explain it and indicate how the profile could be improved, as shown below.

The profile results for the pasta in cheese sauce show that most people thought the following.	The profile could be improved in the following ways.
• It has a poor vegetable flavour.	• Adding fresh or dried herbs to the vegetables • Adding more garlic • Adding red pepper or a little chilli pepper
• It has quite tender vegetables.	This profile is good, so it does not need to be changed.
• The sauce could be smoother.	Making sure that the sauce is properly stirred during cooking and strained at the end to remove any lumps.
• It has quite an attractive colour.	Garnish such as tomato slices and parsley could be added.
• The sauce has quite a cheesy flavour.	This could be improved by using a stronger cheese, such as parmesan or extra mature cheddar.

Recording your results

Keep a record of any tests that you have carried out. This includes keeping the pieces of paper that your testers have written on when they tasted your food. You might be asked to prove that you carried out these tests, and this would be your evidence.

Present the results clearly – a table is a good way of doing this.

Always say how many people tasted the food or how many food products were used in a survey.

Refer to your results when writing up your evaluation.

RECORDING NUTRITIONAL DATA

You may need to support your practical cookery choices for the short tasks with nutritional data. This data will show how much of different nutrients the foods that you make or investigate would have. From this, you could then evaluate the foods in relation to your task. For example, do they provide enough protein or do homemade food products have less fat, salt and sugar than ready-made products?

In the two examples below, nutritional data is asked for in the practical task. In the investigative task you could compare the nutritional value of the ready-made and homemade products when considering the advantages and disadvantages of both.

Practical task	Investigative task
Protein is an important nutrient for the growth, repair and maintenance of the body. Plan and cook two dishes that would provide protein for a person who follows a vegetarian diet. Support your choices with nutritional data. Evaluate your work.	Plan and carry out an investigation into the advantages and disadvantages of using ready-made food products compared to homemade products that use fresh ingredients. Record and display your results, using them as evidence on which to base your conclusions. Evaluate your work.

If you are comparing one food with another, the nutritional data should be given for a standard unit of measurement so that you can make direct comparisons between different food products – give the nutrients found in 100g food or 100mls of liquid.

If you are working out the nutritional value of a recipe, you will need to work out the amount of each nutrient you are investigating in each amount of the ingredients used (an example is shown below).

The nutritional data that you give will depend on the task that you are doing. For the practical task above, only data on the protein content of the dishes would be needed, whereas for the investigative task, you might decide to compare several nutrients such as sodium (salt), fat and sugar.

Finding nutritional data

There are nutritional analysis computer programs available. You input data (the amount of ingredients you are using in a recipe or the amount of a particular dish you are analysing) and are then given a printout of the results for a range of nutrients. Your school or college may have such a program on its computer system.

If there is no computer program available, it is possible to get nutritional data from food composition tables in a book. These tables list a wide variety of foods (they might be listed alphabetically or by groups such as dairy foods, fruits, meat and fish) and show the amount of nutrients they each contain, usually in 100g of food.

Using the practical task example above, the chart on the next page shows how to work out the protein content for each of the ingredients in the pasta with cheese sauce recipe, using food composition tables.

The first column shows you which ingredients are in the recipe and how much of each is used. The second column shows you how much protein there is in 100g of each ingredient (from the food composition tables). The third column shows you how much of each ingredient was used in the recipe. The last column shows you how to work out the protein content for each ingredient.

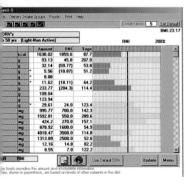

Ingredient	Amount of protein in 100g of ingredient	Amount of ingredient used	How much protein in ingredient used?
Penne pasta	12.0g	200g	12.0g x 2 = 24g
Vegetable oil	0.0g	15g	0g
Garlic	7.9g	10g	7.9g ÷ 10 = 0.79g
Leek	1.6g	75g	1.6g ÷ 100g x 75g = 1.2g
Mushrooms	1.8g	150g	1.8g x 1.5 = 2.7g
Frozen peas	5.7g	100g	5.7g
Butter	0.0g	50g	0g
Plain flour	9.4g	50g	9.4g ÷ 2 = 4.7g
Whole milk	3.2g	500g	3.2g x 5 = 16.0g
Cheddar cheese	25.5g	150g	25.5g x 1.5 = 38.25g
Total amount of protein in pasta with cheese sauce			93.34g

Once you have the total amount of nutrients for the recipe or food, you can work out how many nutrients are in a portion of the food that one person would eat.

In our example, the pasta with cheese sauce recipe contains four portions. The total amount of protein in the recipe is 93.34g. The amount of protein in each portion would therefore be: 93.34 ÷ 4 = 23.3g.

TOPIC

3

EVALUATING YOUR PRACTICAL WORK AND DRAWING CONCLUSIONS

Evaluation is a way of demonstrating what you have understood and learned from carrying out the short task.

A good way to do this is to work your way through each part of the short task (planning, practical and outcome of practical) and make evaluation comments as you go. In this way you are less likely to miss anything out.

To help you to write your evaluation, you may divide it into three parts:
- Identify strengths and weaknesses in all aspects of the short task.
- Suggest or justify improvements to your work.
- Draw conclusions from your work.

Identifying strengths and weaknesses

If you identify weaknesses in your work, it does not mean that you have failed. In fact, it is often quite the opposite. It shows your teacher and examiner that you are aware of the weakness. If you can then suggest how to overcome it, this will demonstrate your understanding of how to improve your work for the next short task.

The table below suggests some strengths and weaknesses that you may identify during or after you have completed your short task.

Possible strengths	Possible weaknesses
You were well organised and worked steadily, which gave you time to present the work properly.	You were disorganised and lost several important pieces of information and results which meant you had to start some of the work all over again.
You completed the work on time, which meant you had time to do it to the best of your ability.	You delayed starting the work, which meant you had to rush the work at the end.
You chose some very suitable practical work which you were able to carry out in the time available and which gave good results. You asked for advice from your teacher to help you with this.	You did not choose your practical work very wisely. Some of the recipes were too complicated and took too long to make in the time available. This was because you did not read them through before you started and did not ask your teacher for advice.
You demonstrated your practical cookery skills very well and produced food that looked very appetising and tasted good. You worked neatly and hygienically and served the food on time.	You had some problems with your practical work and needed some help to complete the practical work on time. The food was not very well served – it was a bit messy and lacked colour and flavour. You had to spend a lot of time afterwards clearing up because you did not work very tidily.
You chose a suitable number of people to taste your work which gave you a good set of results.	You did not ask enough people to taste your work so your results are not very clear or complete.
You presented your results clearly in tables and graphs so it is easy to evaluate them.	Your results were written in words which made them difficult to follow.

Suggesting and justifying improvements to your work

This is an important part of the evaluation process, because it demonstrates that you understand how to:

- make your results more realistic
- improve the standard of your work
- carry out further work to increase your understanding of the subject of the short task.

The table below gives some suggestions of how your work could be improved with justifications for doing so.

Suggestions for improving your work	Justification
Present the work more clearly using headings, sub-headings, charts, diagrams and examples	This makes it easier for an examiner to follow your work and understand what you are trying to explain and demonstrate
Investigate a wider range of food products	This would give you a wider range of results from which to draw conclusions and support what you are trying to prove
Write more detail in your reasons for choice of practical work	This shows that you have really thought through your task and have chosen your practical work carefully
Practise your practical skills	This will help you to work out the recipe you are going to use and to produce a good result. It will also indicate whether you need to make changes to your timed plan.
Be more organised in your practical work – before and during the practical session	This will help you to avoid forgetting something such as an ingredient or an instruction. It will also help you to work efficiently because you will know where everything is and you will not waste time looking for things.
Use a larger number of people to taste your food, or a bigger range of products in a survey	This would make your results more believable and realistic.

Below is an example of how you could write this information (using the practical task example).

- I could have written more in my reasons for choice, e.g. that the dishes can be made in the time available.
- I needed to read the recipes more closely before I started cooking and needed to check that I had all the ingredients. I realised I had forgotten the leek for the pasta with cheese sauce recipe, so I had to use an onion that my teacher had spare instead. This gave flavour but not so much as a leek would have.
- In the practical session I needed to follow my time plan more closely because I forgot to set the oven, so it was not hot enough when my potato layer bake went in which meant it took longer to cook.
- I should have prepared some of the ingredients before the practical session, such as grating the cheese and chopping the vegetables as this would have saved me some time.

- I needed to wash up more during the practical session because I used some equipment that I needed again and it was not ready to use and this wasted time.
- I needed to spend more time on the cheese sauce and less on putting the layers of potato and onion into the dish, which would have made the sauce smoother.
- My cheese sauce was a bit thick when it cooked and slightly lumpy, so I had to stir in some more milk and strain it through a sieve to remove some lumps – this wasted time.
- My potato layer bake looked a bit dull when it came out of the oven, so I put some tomato slices and parsley on it to add colour.
- I should have asked more people to try my dishes as this would have given me a better set of results to evaluate my work.

Drawing conclusions from your work

This section should summarise what you have learned from the short task.

To write a conclusion, you need to do the following:

- go back to the original task title
- decide whether or not the work you have carried out has given you enough information to answer the original question
- explain what you have learned about the short task topic and how what you have done has increased your understanding of the topic.

Using our original examples, the charts below give some suggestions about what you could write in your conclusion:

Practical task

Protein is an important nutrient for the growth, repair and maintenance of the body.

Plan and cook two dishes that would provide protein for a person who follows a vegetarian diet. Support your choices with nutritional data.

Evaluate your work.

Suggested main course dishes:

- pasta with cheese sauce
- vegetable lasagne
- tomato and cheese pizza
- vegetable curry with chickpeas
- lentil dhal.

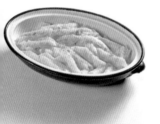

Conclusions

In this task I was asked to plan and cook dishes that would provide enough protein for a vegetarian. I think my choices were good because when I did the nutritional analysis, I found that a portion of the pasta with cheese sauce provided enough protein to supply about a third of the amount an adult needs each day.

Everyone who tasted the dishes said they liked them, although the pasta dish was liked more, probably because of the sauce. Some of the people who tried the dishes were vegetarian, and they said that the dishes were very nice and tasty. I was pleased about this as this was the whole point of the task.

My task has shown that it is possible to make interesting and tasty vegetarian food using simple ingredients like pasta and lentils, and also to provide enough protein using ingredients such as milk and cheese. So I think I have answered the task quite well.

Investigative task

Plan and carry out an investigation into the advantages and disadvantages of using ready-made food products compared to homemade products that use fresh ingredients. Record and display your results, using them as evidence on which to base your conclusions.

Evaluate your work.

Suggested ready-made food products that you could compare with homemade versions:

- cottage pie
- curry
- soups
- savoury flans (quiche)
- pasties
- cheesecake.

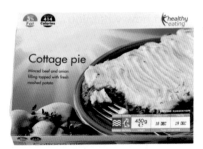

Ready-made cottage pie

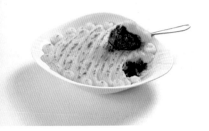

Homemade cottage pie

Conclusions:

In this task I was asked to look at the advantages and disadvantages of buying ready-made food compared to homemade food. I decided that the best way to do this was to compare the same type of foods and so I chose to compare ready-made cottage pies with a homemade version. I looked at the fat and salt content, the price and the time they took to prepare.

I found that the ready-made cottage pies were quite high in salt and fat compared to my homemade one, although this was not picked up by the tasting panel. This showed me that people can eat fat and salt without really realising it, and that you can cut these down in homemade food by using lean meat and not adding salt. Also, by making meals like this yourself, you can decide exactly what goes into it.

I was surprised by how much packaging was used in the ready-made cottage pies, and this added to the cost. Also, the servings were quite small, so although they seemed to cost less, there was actually a lot less to eat than the homemade version. The cost of the ready-made cottage pies varied quite a lot, and the most expensive one was rated lower for flavour and texture than some of the cheaper ones. The homemade version made enough for three meals and it could be frozen easily, which would save money and time.

The ready-made cottage pies were very easy and quick to cook, which would save people time if they are busy, so I could understand why they are popular. The homemade version took a lot longer to prepare and cook, but if you make a lot of it in one go and freeze it, you would save time.

Everyone liked my homemade cottage pie and they liked most of the ready-made ones.

I think I answered the task well because I compared several ready-made cottage pies with my homemade one. I was able to conclude that ready-made foods have advantages in saving time for some people because of their busy lifestyle, but that it is also easy to make a homemade version that has better ingredients in it and can save money.

PRESENTATION OF WORK AND USE OF ICT

Once you have completed your short tasks you will be asked to present them for your teacher and the examination board to assess.

Whether you handwrite your work or use a computer to wordprocess it, you should spend time making sure that it is presented clearly and neatly. This will create a good impression and make it easy for your teacher and an examiner to understand what you have done.

The short tasks should each have the following sections:

- A title page showing your name, candidate number and centre number (your teacher will tell you what these numbers are) and the title of your short task.
- Your work, divided up into:
  - how you planned the short task
  - what you did for your practical work, including reasons for choice, recipes, timed plans
  - the results of your taste testing, surveys and costings
  - the evaluation of your work
  - your conclusions.
- A list of references you have used (books, magazines and journals, internet pages, TV programmes).

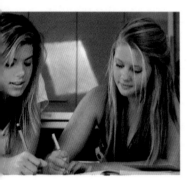

Each section should have a title and you should make use of headings and sub-headings to set out your work clearly. Where possible, support your work with photographs of practical work, taste testing panels and surveys you have carried out.

If you have word processed your work on a computer, you may be required to save your work for each short task electronically in a 'controlled assessment portfolio'. This is a collection of folders and files containing your work and it forms the evidence for your assessment.

Your teacher will explain and show you how to organise your folders effectively on your school intranet. Each file and folder should have a name.

If you use a computer for your work, it is very important that you back up your work by making a copy of it, for example on a USB memory stick. In this way, if there is a problem with retrieving your work at school, you will be able to produce a copy.

INTRODUCTION

During your GCSE Food and Nutrition course you will be expected to complete one food study task. You will carry this out over a period of time (your teacher will tell you how long) and it will involve research and practical work.

You will be given a set of food study themes to choose from and your teacher will help you choose the most suitable one for you. Once you have chosen a theme, you will need to develop a suitable and manageable task title, which your teacher will also help you with.

During the food study task you must produce a log of practical work. This is a record of all the practical work you make during the task and is used as evidence for your final grade. More details about this are given later.

The aim of the food study task is for you to demonstrate your ability to carry out research into a topic of particular interest to you and to plan and carry out suitable practical work to support your research. The chart below explains how you will be assessed.

How you will be assessed	Which knowledge and skills the food study task will test you on
Research	• How you justify your choice of food study theme and task title • How you identify the sources of information you will use to research this theme and title • How you carry out primary and secondary research • How you present your research results and draw conclusions from them
Selecting and planning practical tasks	• How you use your research results to produce a list of suitable ideas for practical work • How you sort and assess your ideas • How you select suitable final choices for your practical work • How you select other activities to support your work e.g. leaflets, displays, tasting panels • How you justify your final choices of practical work • How you produce plans (timed plans, ingredients lists) for your chosen practical work • How you plan and record evidence of your practical work
Practical work	• How well you follow your timed plan of work and make use of the time available • How well and effectively you organise your work space, equipment and ingredients • How cleanly and tidily you work and your attention to food hygiene • How safely and independently you use kitchen equipment • How many different cooking methods you use and how well you use them • How many types of skills you demonstrate, including practical cookery skills, ICT skills, costing and taste testing

▶

How you will be assessed	Which knowledge and skills the food study task will test you on
Outcomes of the practical work	• How well you complete your log of practical work • The quality of the practical work you make and how well you present it • How well you carry out some tasting panels for your practical work and how accurately you record the results
Evaluation of the task	• Your ability to review your work and identify the strengths and weaknesses of all aspects of your completed food study task • Your ability to suggest how you could improve the work, with reasons • What conclusions you have drawn from the food study task • How well you present your written work

The following example is used to explain how to carry out the food study task so that you understand what to do.

Food study task

Theme: Healthy eating

Title: There has been a large rise in the sales of ready meals and takeaway meals. Investigate the reasons for this and the probable health implications. How successfully can these popular fast meals be prepared at home from fresh ingredients?

TOPIC 1

RESEARCH

CHOOSING A FOOD STUDY THEME

Your first job is to choose a food study theme from the list that your teacher will give you.

Choose one theme that you are the most interested in and the one that you could find out enough information about.

Choosing and producing a task title

Once you have made your decision, you need to start to produce a task title.

Here is some advice to help you produce a task title:

● Make notes of the various topics your chosen theme covers. Using our example theme (Healthy eating), this is what you could write.

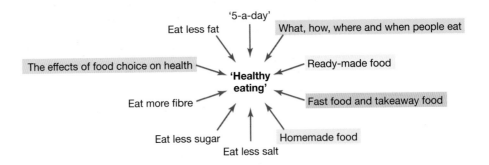

Decide which of the topics you want to include in your research. In the example, the ones which will be included are highlighted.

Produce a task title that indicates what type of practical work you are going to do. The example title below is highlighted to show where each of the topics above fits into it.

> There has been a large rise in the sales of ready meals and takeaway meals. Investigate the reasons for this and the probable health implications.
>
> How successfully can these popular fast meals be prepared at home from fresh ingredients?

Justifying your choice of study task

The next job is to justify (give reasons) for your choice of study theme and title. Using the example, you could give reasons such as:

- Healthy eating is an important theme because many people are concerned about the effects of what they eat on their health.
- Eating habits have changed over the years and at the same time the numbers of people with diet-related health conditions (obesity and heart disease) have increased, so it would be interesting to investigate if there is a link between these.
- There are lots of different types of ready meals and takeaway meals to choose from for the investigation.
- Many people need to save money when buying food, so the practical work will attempt to demonstrate that you can make homemade versions of popular foods that are tasty, economical and also of benefit to health.

CARRYING OUT RESEARCH

Identifying sources of information

The next job is to identify the sources of information you will use to research this theme and title. In the example you could use any of the following:

- the internet, newspaper and magazine articles for information on diet-related diseases and the numbers of ready-made and takeaway meals that are bought and eaten
- a survey of your nearest town to find out the number of fast food outlets
- a survey of your local supermarket to find out the types and numbers of ready-made meals sold
- a survey of the nutritional value of ready-made and fast food products compared to homemade versions, using a nutritional analysis computer program.

Carrying out research

The next job is to carry out your primary and secondary research.

SECONDARY RESEARCH

Secondary research is about gathering information from books, the internet, newspaper and magazine articles and journals. It is used to support your primary research and help you to give examples.

When you are carrying out secondary research, there are a few important rules that you must follow:

- Be very selective about which information you use – only use information that is directly to do with your food study task.
- You should write out the information that you find from secondary research in your own words. You are not allowed to directly copy other people's work and call it your own.
- If you collect information from the internet, DO NOT copy and paste the information into your work. You will be found out as copied and pasted work is very easy to detect. You must write everything in your own words.
- Information that you use from secondary research has been written by someone else, so you must acknowledge this by showing at the end of your work where the information came from. This is called referencing your work.
- At the end of your food study task you should include a page of references (sometimes called a bibliography). This lists all the books, internet sites, magazine and journal articles that you have used in your secondary research.

For a book you would list it as shown here:

Author family name and initial of first name, year of publication, title of book (in *italics*), name of publisher, where it was published (city), e.g:

Blythman, J. (2006) *Bad Food Britain – how a nation ruined its appetite,* Fourth Estate, London

For a magazine article:

Who wrote the article, the year it was published, the title of the article (in quotes), the magazine title (in italics), more details about the issue and month of publication, the pages where the article appeared, e.g:

The Food Commission, (2008) 'Fast food chains under pressure to label menus', *The Food Magazine,* Issue 83, October/December, p. 4

For an article found on the internet:

Who wrote the article, the date or year the article was written, the title of the article, the website page reference, e.g:

Which? magazine, (2008) *'What's really in takeaway food',* http://www.which.co.uk/advice/whats-really-in-takeaway-food/index.jsp

PRIMARY RESEARCH

Primary research is research that you design and carry out yourself. You collect results from it that you can then discuss and draw conclusions from. It includes activities such as those shown in the chart below, using the example.

Types of primary reseach	Examples
Surveys	How often people eat fast or takeaway foods
	The types of fast or takeaway foods they eat
	The number and types of fast food and takeaway shops and restaurants in a town
	A survey of ready-made meals to find out about the cost, ingredients, portion sizes and nutritional value
Questionnaires	Ask a range of people to fill in a questionnaire about their shopping and eating habits and if and how they have changed
Interviews	Ask an elderly relative or friend to recall how they used to grow, buy, prepare and cook their food and what they used to eat and how it is different to now
TV programme or film reviews	Watch some documentary programmes or films about the effects of eating fast food on health
	Summarise and review what you have seen
Shop visits	To find out the range of fast and ready-made foods sold
	To find out how shops sell ready-made foods
	To find out how many types of fast foods and ready-made meals they sell

▶

Types of primary reseach	Examples
Letters to food companies	• To find out which types of foods they sell are the most popular • To find out if they provide any nutritional information about their food products
Case studies	• Record and analyse the shopping, cooking and eating habits of a family for a week (ask the family to keep a food diary) • Invite them to try your food products and give their opinions about them
Food tasting and testing	• Ask a group of people to taste and score your food products on a range of sensory qualities (see page 12)

> *Warning: Food companies receive lots of letters from students studying for exams. Make sure that you ask them a question so that they can easily answer you. For example, 'Which types of ready-made meals that you make or sell are the most popular?'*
>
> *If you ask a very general question such as 'Can you send me some information on the food you sell' it will be more difficult for them to answer.*

You should carry out one or two pieces of primary research as follows:

- State the aim of your research. For example, 'I am going to carry out a survey of ready-made meals in my local supermarket to find out the types of meals that are sold and what ingredients they contain to help me choose which ones to prepare as home made.'
- Plan and carry out the research carefully and thoroughly. For example, for a survey, prepare some charts or tables before you do the survey that you can fill in quickly and easily. This will help you to analyse the information.
- Present the results of your research in the form of a table or chart so it is easy for an examiner to see what you did and how you have used the information.

Writing a questionnaire

Questionnaires are commonly used in primary research to find out information about what people do or what their opinion is about something. They need to be carefully designed so that they:

- are not too complicated – the questions need to be simple and the text should be easy to read
- do not take a long time to answer
- are easy to follow – whole questions are on the same page and not split up
- give you the information you are looking for.

A questionnaire should be set out as follows:

1 The aim of the questionnaire – tell people what the questionnaire is about and why you are asking them to take part.
2 A statement to tell people that their answers will be confidential (their names will not be used).
3 Simple instructions about how to complete your questionnaire ('tick the box' or 'write your answer in the space provided').
4 Start with easy questions first, such as 'Are you male/female?' and 'What age group are you?'
5 Continue with questions about the information you are trying to find out.

There are two types of questions:

- Closed questions are ones in which people are asked to choose one of a list of possible answers that the question gives them, such as yes or no, I agree strongly/I agree/I neither agree nor disagree/I disagree/I disagree strongly' or I liked it a lot/I liked it/I neither liked nor disliked it/I disliked it/I disliked it a lot. You can use the 'Smiley' face symbols to help explain this.

  Closed questions are useful because they only take a little time to answer. They also give definite information to the person doing the research. Another advantage is that you do not have to read someone's handwriting. They must be carefully designed so that the questions are easily understood and all the information you want to find out is covered.

- Open questions are ones where the person filling out the questionnaire can answer in any way they want. For example, you might ask, 'What do you think about...?', 'What is your opinion about...?' or 'What do you think is the best thing about...?'

  Open questions are useful because you usually get a true opinion or attitude from the answer, but they do take longer to complete and some people may not bother to answer them or will give an unhelpful answer.

Most questionnaires are a mixture of both types of questions. Here is an example of a questionnaire that could be used for the food study task.

Your help is needed for some research about eating ready meals and takeaway food. *You do not have to put your name on the questionnaire.*

Please read the following questions and fill in the boxes as requested. It should only take a few minutes to complete. Please return your completed survey to your tutor.

1. This question is about you. Please tick the boxes which apply to you.

   How old are you?   11–13 years ☐   14–16 years ☐   17–19 years ☐

   Are you Male ☐   Female ☐

2. How often do you eat a ready-made meal bought from a supermarket?

   Never ☐   About once a month ☐   At least once a week ☐

   More than once a week ☐   Every day ☐

3. How often do you eat a takeaway meal bought from a fast food outlet?

   Never ☐   About once a month ☐   At least once a week ☐

   More than once a week ☐   Every day ☐

4. Put the following ready meals and takeaway meals in the order in which you like them by putting a number in the boxes where 1 = your most favourite and 6 = your least favourite.

Ready meals		Takeaway meals	
Curries	☐	Fish and chips	☐
Meat or vegetable pies and pasties	☐	Indian food	☐
Chinese food	☐	Burgers and fries	☐
Pasta meals e.g. lasagne	☐	Chinese food	☐
Soups	☐	Fried chicken	☐
Fish dishes (fish cakes or fish in a sauce)	☐	Kebabs	☐

5. Why do you think ready-made meals and takeaway foods are so popular?

   _____

   _____

Thank you for your help

RESULTS AND CONCLUSIONS

The final job in this section is to present your research results and draw conclusions from them.

The results of your primary research can be presented in a number of ways, as for the short tasks (see page 21).

If you have collected data from a survey or questionnaire, you could present the results as one of the following:

- graph
- bar chart
- pie chart
- table of results – numbers, percentages or fractions
- a written account (for an interview).

HANDLING AND USING NUTRITIONAL DATA

For your food study task you may have decided to investigate the nutritional value of the foods you are going to make or are going to compare to ready-made foods.

It is possible to use nutritional analysis computer programs for this purpose, and your school or college may have one on its computer system that you can use. If you do not have the use of a program, you can find out the data in books that contain tables of nutrients for different foods.

When you have collected the nutritional information, you need to know how to make the best use of it for your food study task. The example below will help to explain what to do.

The first thing to do is to collect the nutritional data.

On the next page is the data from a computer nutrient analyser program for 100g of homemade chicken korma curry (in the middle) and 100g of ready-made chicken korma curry (on the right).

The measurements used are:

mcg = microgram (1/1,000,000 of a gram)
mg = milligram (1/1,000 of a gram)
g = gram (1/1,000 of a kilogram)

You will see that the program gives you lots of nutritional data, only some of which you may want to use. In the example food study task, the fat and salt content of takeaway and ready-made foods could be compared with homemade versions, so these nutrients have been highlighted on the table in pink.

It would also be interesting to compare some other nutrients, such as protein, iron and vitamin C as well as fibre and water. These have been highlighted in green.

By comparing 100g of homemade curry with 100g of ready-made curry, you make a direct comparison between them, and can talk about the nutrients as percentages. For example, in the data above the homemade curry has 15.2 per cent protein and 5.8 per cent fat, whereas the ready-made curry has 12.0 per cent protein and 17.0 per cent fat.

This also makes it easy to compare these figures with the dietary reference values (DRVs) (see page 87) for different people and comment on how much a food product would contribute towards these DRVs.

ACTIVITY

With reference to the sample questionnaire above.

a) Which of the questions are closed questions?
b) Which are open questions?
c) Using the sample food study task, write two closed and two open questions of your own and try them out on some one in your class to see what sort of answers you get.
d) Which types of question are easier to present the results of?

ACTIVITY

Look at the two sets of nutritional data in the chart on the next page, and answer these questions.

1 Which one has the most protein?
2 Which one has the most fat?
3 Which one has the most sodium?
4 Which one is the most energy dense?
5 Which one has the most fibre?

Nutrient	Amount in 100g ready made curry	Amount in 100g homemade curry
kcals	222	130
kJ	932	547
Protein	12.0g	15.20g
Fat	17.0g	5.80g
Carbohydrate	6.0g	4.6g
Iron	800mcg	800mcg
Magnesium	27mg	27mg
Calcium	61mg	61mg
Zinc	700mcg	700mcg
Iodine	11.00mcg	11.00mcg
Sodium	0.8g	0.2g
Vitamin B1	98mcg	100mcg
Vitamin B2	100mcg	120mcg
Vitamin B3	5mcg	5mcg
Vitamin B6	270mcg	280mcg
Vitamin B9	6.00mcg	7.00mcg
Vitamin B12	0	0
Vitamin C	0g	1mg
Vitamin A	15mcg	18mcg
Vitamin D	0.8mcg	0.10mcg
Vitamin E	125mcg	130mcg
Fibre	370mg	500mg
Water	78.0g	71.40g

Once you have analysed your homemade foods, you could suggest some ways of changing the levels of some of the nutrients, as shown in the examples below.

Nutrient	Problem	What could be changed?
Protein	Too low	Increase meat, fish, egg, milk, beans or cheese content
Fat	Too high	• Change the cooking method from frying to grilling or oven baking • Reduce the fat content by 50 per cent and try the finished result to see if it makes much difference to the taste and texture • Use reduced fat versions of some ingredients
Salt	Too high	• Use alternative flavours such as herbs • Change some of the ingredients that may contain salt
Sugar	Too high	• Reduce the added sugar content by 50 per cent and try the finished result to see if it makes much difference to the taste and texture • Try using naturally sweet foods such as fruits or carrots instead of added sugar
Fibre	Too low	Add more fruits, vegetables or use wholegrain cereals

You then need to present your nutritional data clearly (as a chart or graph) so that your teacher or examiner can understand what you have used it for.

TOPIC 2

PLANNING AND CARRYING OUT PRACTICAL TASKS

PLANNING PRACTICAL TASKS

Having carried out your research, your next main job is to plan your practical tasks to support what you have already found out. You have to do a minimum of four practical tasks, of which at least three are practical food tasks and possibly one can be a non-food supporting activity.

Going back to the food study task title again, the practical work is in the second part of the title, as shown below.

> There has been a large rise in the sales of ready meals and takeaway meals. Investigate the reasons for this and the probable health implications. How successfully can these popular fast meals be prepared at home from fresh ingredients?

This is what you must do.

Using your research findings, write down what your practical work is aiming to demonstrate or prove.

Ideas for practical work

Make a list of suitable ideas for practical work. Using the example, here are some suggestions.

Types of products	Suggested practical work
Takeaway foods	• Burgers – meat and vegetarian • Homemade burger buns • Chicken nuggets – oven baked, not fried • Kebabs – meat and vegetarian
Ready-made meals	• Curry – chicken and vegetarian • Sweet and sour Chinese pork or chicken and vegetarian alternative (tofu or Quorn) • Meat pie – beef or chicken • Pasta with a sauce

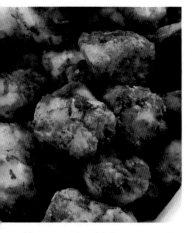

Homemade chicken nuggets

Sort and assess your suggested ideas, using some of the following ideas:
- Work out how much time they will take to prepare and cook – can you complete them in your lesson time?
- How much will the ingredients cost?
- Do you know how to make the recipes? Can you practise them?
- Carry out a nutritional assessment of your recipes using a computer program (see later) compared to the nutritional information from the manufacturers of ready-made or fast foods – how does your homemade version compare? Does it have less fat, salt or sugar?
- Make some of your recipes in some of your lessons, ask people to taste them and give their opinions.

Choose recipes

Once you have decided which recipes are the most suitable, choose a minimum of three (or four if no non-food supporting activity is chosen), referring to your research results and justifying your reasons for choice (see page 7).

Using the example, here are some reasons for the choices made.

Chosen recipe	Reasons for choice
Homemade beef burger	• Very popular takeaway food • Easy and quick to prepare using a food processor • Can be oven baked or grilled • Can have a variety of flavours added, such as pepper, ginger, garlic, herbs or chilli, to make it more interesting • Quite economical to make • Vegetables and breadcrumbs can be added to the meat to lower the cost
Homemade vegetarian burger	• As above, but using beans, vegetables and nuts in the mixture • May need to be fried to add moisture but could be oven baked – not grilled
Chicken nuggets	• Very popular takeaway food • Can be made with lean chicken breast meat which improves the protein content • Can have a variety of flavours added, such as pepper, ginger, garlic, herbs or chilli, to make it more interesting • Can be oven baked • Easy and quick to prepare using the food processor
Chicken curry	• Very popular ready-made meal • Quite economical to make – especially if a whole chicken is bought and jointed rather than buying ready-cut chicken joints • Easy and quick to prepare – can be cooked in a pan on the hob or in the oven while other practical activity is going on • Can be frozen in bulk for future meals so saves time and adds convenience
Lentil and vegetable curry	• As above, but a variety of vegetables used • Very economical if vegetables are in season and purchased from a market
Pasta with cheese and vegetable sauce	• Pasta is very economical to buy • Very quick to prepare • Can be frozen in bulk so saves time • A variety of vegetables can be used • Very economical if vegetables are in season and purchased from a market • Flavourings, such as herbs, garlic or nutmeg, can be used to vary the flavour

NON-FOOD SUPPORTING ACTIVITY

You might choose to carry out a non-food supporting activity as part of your practical tasks. Here are some ideas:

- A tasting panel (see page 12) to compare your homemade products with some bought ready-made products – ask tasters to rate or profile your finished results.

- A display of the cost and ingredients of your homemade recipes compared to a range of shop bought products.
- A PowerPoint presentation about your food study task.
- A leaflet of recipes you have made.

OTHER FORMS OF EVIDENCE

Produce timed plans of your practical work (see page 9) and comment on them when you have finished the work:

- Were you able to prepare the work within the time you had?
- Have you been able to demonstrate that homemade food does not take very long to make?

Produce lists of ingredients that you will use in your practical work, and comment on them when you have finished the work:

- Were the ingredients suitable for the task?
- Did people like the ingredients you used?
- Would or could you have changed any of the ingredients and why?

You must record evidence of your practical work. You could use:

- a digital camera and record the pictures in your write-up of your work
- charts, rating scales, radar diagrams (see page 13) for your tasting panel results.

PRACTICAL WORK AND OUTCOMES

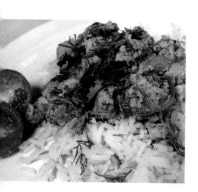

Practical work

In your food study task, whenever you carry out a practical food preparation and cooking activity, you should demonstrate the following:

- How well you follow your timed plan of work and make use of the time available.
- How well and effectively you organise your work space, equipment and ingredients.
- How cleanly and tidily you work and your attention to food hygiene.
- How safely and independently you use kitchen equipment.
- How many different cooking methods you use and how well you use them.
- How many types of skills you demonstrate, including practical cookery skills, ICT skills, costing and taste testing.

The importance of organising your resources effectively and using equipment safely, effectively and independently has already been covered in Unit B001 (see pages 10–11).

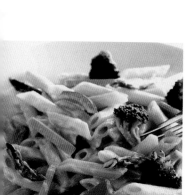

Outcomes of the practical work

You must make sure that the standard of the completed practical work you produce is the best you can do. You should pay particular attention to the following:

- the presentation of your practical work – does it look appetising, neat, colourful, appropriately garnished, cooked just right, well served?
- the flavour of the food – have you tasted it and adjusted the flavour before you serve it?
- the texture of the food – have you cooked the food thoroughly, so that it is safe to eat but not overcooked?

You must also make sure that you carefully and neatly record all your results from your tasting panels, practical log (see example on next page) and photographs, so that they can support your practical work.

Date	Type of practical activity	Work completed	Skills demonstrated	Teacher verification
14 Sep	Cooking and photograph work Taste panel	Chicken curry	Prepared chicken breasts Prepared a range of vegetables Prepared curry sauce	
21 Sep	Cooking and photograph work Taste panel	Pasta with cheese and vegetable sauce	Vegetable preparation Sauce making	
28 Sep	Recipe leaflet	Introduction and first two recipes completed		
5 Oct	Cooking and photograph work Taste panel	Homemade beef burger and vegetarian burger	Use of food processor Shaping of burgers	

TOPIC 3

EVALUATION AND DRAWING CONCLUSIONS FROM YOUR WORK

EVALUATION OF YOUR PRACTICAL RESULTS

Evaluation is a way of demonstrating what you have understood and learned from carrying out the food study task. You can make evaluation comments throughout your work, but you should also include them all together in this section.

You could evaluate each of the sections of your food study task in turn:
- Section 1: Research
- Section 2: Selecting and planning your practical tasks
- Section 3: Practical work
- Section 4: Outcomes of your practical work

For each of these sections you need to do the following:
- Identify strengths and weaknesses in all aspects of the food study task.
- Refer to and justify improvements or changes that you made to your work.

Identifying strengths and weaknesses

If you identify weaknesses in your work, it does not mean that you have failed. In fact it is often quite the opposite. It shows your teacher and examiner that you are aware of the weakness, and if you were able to suggest how it could be overcome, this will demonstrate your understanding of how you were able to improve your work.

The table below suggests some strengths and weaknesses that you may identify during or after you have completed your food study task.

Possible strengths	Possible weaknesses
Section 1: Research	
You were well organised and carried out the work steadily, which gave you time to present the work properly	You were disorganised and lost several important pieces of information and results which meant you had to start some of the work all over again
You completed the work on time, which meant you had time to complete the work to the best of your ability	You delayed starting the work, which meant you had to rush the work at the end
You produced a focused task title and were able to give reasons for your choice	Your task title was rather open ended and this made it difficult to focus on what to research
You identified a good range of sources of information for your research and were able to use them effectively	You could not find enough information and should have spent more time on this part of the task
You carried out a range of primary research methods which gave you some good results on which to base your practical work	You didn't carry out enough primary research and so had limited results from which to choose your practical work
You used a range of secondary research which gave you some useful information to write about	You used a limited range of secondary research and found it difficult to find any more
Section 2: Selecting and planning your practical tasks	
You chose some very suitable practical work which you were able to carry out in the time available and which gave good results. You asked for advice from your teacher to help you with this	You did not choose your practical work very wisely – some of the recipes were too complicated and took too long to make in the time available. This was because you did not read them through before you started and did not ask your teacher for advice

▶

Possible strengths	Possible weaknesses
Section 3: Practical work	
You were well organised and worked carefully and tidily and were able to complete the work on time	You were rather disorganised and realised you had forgotten to bring some ingredients, which meant that you had to use a different ingredient that was available
	You did not clear up as you worked which meant you had a lot to do at the end of the practical lesson
	You had to rush your work because you ran out of time
Section 4: Outcomes of your practical work	
You chose a suitable number of people to taste your work which gave you a good set of results	You did not ask enough people to taste your work so your results are not very clear or complete
You presented your results clearly in tables and graphs so it is easy to evaluate them	Your results were written in words which made them difficult to follow

Suggesting or justifying improvements

This is an important part of the evaluation process, because it demonstrates that you understand how to:

- make your results more realistic
- improve the standard of your work
- carry out further work to increase your understanding of the subject of the food study task.

Suggestions for improving your work	Justification
Section 1: Research	
Present the work more clearly using headings, sub-headings, charts, diagrams and examples	This makes it easier for an examiner to follow your work and understand what you are trying to explain and demonstrate.
Use a wider range of sources of information rather than just the internet	This would give you more ideas, examples and information to support what you are investigating.
Investigate a wider range of food products	This would give you a wider range of results from which to draw conclusions and support what you are trying to prove.
Section 2: Selecting and planning your practical tasks	
Spend more time on the secondary research	This would improve your understanding of the study task theme and help you to focus your research and practical work. Get advice from your teacher about what you can make in the time available. This will help make sure that you have enough time to complete your practical tasks.
Section 3: Practical work	
Practise the recipes first	This will build your confidence and ensure that what you plan to make can be made in the time available. Get everything ready the night before the practical lesson. This will help to make sure that you do not forget anything when you are rushing to leave in the morning.
Section 4: Outcomes of your practical work	
Use a larger number of people to taste your food or a bigger range of products in a survey	This would make your results more believable and realistic.

The table gives some suggestions of how your work could be improved with justifications for doing so.

Once you have identified strengths and weaknesses in each section of your work and have suggested improvements, you then need to draw conclusions from what you have done and suggest further work that you could do.

DRAWING CONCLUSIONS FROM YOUR WORK

Drawing (bringing together) conclusions from your work is the final stage of the food study task, and its purpose is to draw together (bring together) all you have learned from the process and give it a neat finish.

To do this, you need to do the following:
- Summarise what you have learned from the food study task.
- Go back to the original study task title and decide whether or not the work you have carried out has given you enough information to answer it.
- Explain what you have learned about the study task theme and how what you have done has increased your understanding of it.

Using the example food study task, the following conclusions might be drawn.
- It is possible to make homemade versions of many popular takeaway and ready-made foods quite easily.
- Most recipes took little time and effort to make, apart from the pasta and cheese sauce recipe which resulted in quite a lot of clearing up which added time to the process.
- All the homemade versions were enjoyed by most of the taste testers.
- The results of the nutritional analysis of the homemade versions showed that they contained less fat, salt and sugar than the ready-made and takeaway foods, which is better for long-term health.
- Making the homemade versions made me and the taste testers realise what types of ingredients are put in to commercially produced ready-made and takeaway foods. It has made some of us decide to prepare our own foods at home and cut down on how much ready-made food we eat, because we prefer to know what is in our food.

Suggesting further work
This section will show the teacher and examiner that you are able to think widely about your food study task theme and can show that you are aware that more research could be done. For the example you could make suggestions such as:
- Use a wider range of foods to compare homemade versions with – baby foods, cakes, desserts, salads and breads.
- Show how basic recipes for breads, sauces, meat dishes and desserts can be adapted to make them healthier by using different ingredients and cooking methods.

TOPIC

1

FUNCTION AND ROLE OF NUTRIENTS

THE MAIN MACRO AND MICRONUTRIENTS IN THE DIET

Our bodies are like very complicated machines. They need energy (fuel) and materials to build, maintain and repair them and to make them work properly and keep going for a long time. We eat food to provide all the energy and materials that our bodies need. These materials are called nutrients and nutrition is the study of them.

There are different types of nutrients and they are put into two groups:

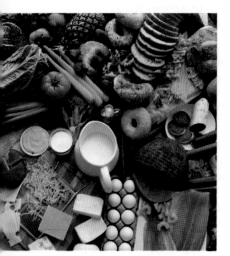

- Macronutrients: These are needed by the body in large amounts and they are protein, fat and carbohydrate.
- Micronutrients: These are needed by the body in small amounts and they are vitamins, minerals and trace elements.

You will also learn about other important materials and natural substances in foods which are important for health. These are:

- **water**: found naturally in foods and as a drink
- **fibre**: found naturally in plant foods.

What else is in food?

Apart from nutrients, water and fibre there are other substances in foods. They include:

- flavourings and colourings: these may be found naturally in the food or added by a food manufacturer to processed food
- enzymes: these are natural chemicals which cause foods such as fruits to become ripe or to break down once they are harvested
- preservatives: these may be found naturally in the food (e.g. acids) or added by a food manufacturer to processed food
- substances that give texture: such as 'stone' cells that give pears a gritty texture or carrageen (from seaweed) which gives a smooth texture for milk products such as yogurt.

ASSESSMENT FOR LEARNING

Here is a picture of the nutritional information on a food label.

1 Which macronutrients and micronutrients are listed on this food label?
2 Why do you think this information is put on food labels?

Nutrition information			
Typical values	**Per 100g**	**Per 30g serving**	**% based on GDA for women**
Energy	2325 kJ	698 kJ	
	559 kcal	168 kcal	8.4%
Protein	**0.2g**	trace	trace
Carbohydrate	**46.3g**	13.9g	6.0%
of which **sugars**	**46.3g**	13.9g	15.4%
Fat	**38.8g**	11.6g	16.6%
of which **saturates**	**25.4g**	7.6g	38.0%
Fibre	**nil**	nil	nil
Salt	**trace**	trace	trace
of which **sodium**	trace	trace	trace

DIETS

What is a diet? Many people think that the word 'diet' means trying to lose weight. This is not quite true because the correct definition of a diet is 'the food that you eat every day'. So everyone is on a diet! Sometimes people have to follow a special diet to improve their health in some way, so they might follow one of the following diets:

- a weight loss diet
- a fat reduced diet
- a low salt diet
- a high fibre diet.

What should we eat?

In order to grow, stay healthy and have enough energy we should eat a variety of foods every day. This is because different foods contain different amounts and types of nutrients. We should aim to have a balanced diet. This means eating the right amounts of nutrients from a variety of foods every day for our particular needs.

As we go through life, our needs for nutrients change. When we are babies, children and teenagers, we are growing fast and so we need a balanced diet to allow this to happen as well as to repair our bodies when we damage them.

When we become adults we need the right foods to maintain and repair the body. During pregnancy and when breastfeeding a baby, women need extra nutrients to enable their bodies to cope with the demands of the growing baby. As people get older they need a balanced diet to continue to maintain and repair their bodies, but they gradually need less energy as their bodies slow down.

Malnutrition means 'bad' nutrition, when the body has either too much of some nutrients (e.g. fat) or not enough, and suffers as a result.

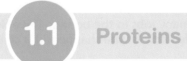

1.1   Proteins

WHAT ARE PROTEINS?

Protein is a macronutrient. Why does the body need it?

- Protein makes the body grow.
- Protein maintains the body to keep it working well.
- Protein repairs the body if it is damaged.
- Protein can also give the body some energy.

Proteins are very big molecules and they are made up of small units called amino acids. There are many different amino acids which mix together in different numbers and formations to produce lots of different proteins.

Some amino acids are essential for children and adults and they must be provided ready-made by the protein in food. All the other amino acids that children and adults need do not have to be ready-made and can be put together inside the body from the protein eaten in food.

Protein foods that contain all of the essential amino acids are said to have high biological value (HBV). Protein foods that are missing one or more essential amino acids are said to have low biological value (LBV). If a mixture of these LBV proteins is eaten every day, all the essential amino acids will be provided, so they are good sources of protein.

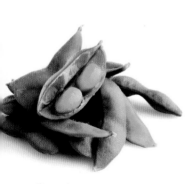

Soya beans

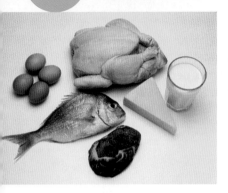

HBV sources of protein

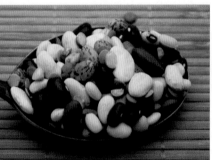

Beans and lentils

ACTIVITY

1 Give three reasons why our bodies need protein.
2 What is the name of the small units that make up proteins?
3 What is meant by high biological value (HBV) protein?
4 What is meant by low biological value (LBV) protein?
5 Name five foods that are good HBV sources of protein.
6 Name three foods that are good LBV sources of protein.
7 Name the protein that is found in wheat.
8 Name the protein that is found in meat.

Which foods give us protein?

These foods are HBV sources of protein:

- milk
- meat
- fish
- cheese
- eggs
- soya beans.

These foods are LBV sources of protein:

- cereals (rice, wheat millet, oats, quinoa)
- peas, beans (except soya beans) and lentils
- nuts and seeds.

Protein names

Foods are made up of different proteins. Each type of protein has a name.

Some examples of protein names are:

- ovalbumin: found in egg white
- gluten: found in wheat
- collagen: found in meat
- caseinogen: found in cheese
- lactoglobulin: found in milk

How much protein do we need?

Everyone needs to have protein every day, but the amount that is needed will change during our lives as we grow, become adults and change our life styles and activities.

Babies, children and teenagers need more protein for their body size than adults to allow for their body growth as well as everything else that protein is needed for. Adults, who have stopped growing, need protein to maintain and repair their body and to grow their hair, finger nails and replace body cells (e.g. red blood cells). Pregnant and lactating (breastfeeding) women need extra protein to allow for the development of the baby.

Protein is needed for many jobs in the body so if we do not have enough, the body will begin to suffer. This is what happens if a child does not have enough protein:

- They stop growing.
- Their hair becomes very thin.
- They cannot digest food properly.
- They have diarrhoea.
- They catch infections easily.
- Fluid builds up under their skin (this is called oedema).
- They become very thin and weak.

This is what happens if an adult does not have enough protein:

- They lose fat and muscle from their body.
- Their internal organs become weak.
- Their hair and skin become dry.
- They get oedema.

It is very rare to see protein deficiency in developed countries like the UK.

If we have too much protein in our diet, it makes the liver and kidneys work harder because they have to process the protein in the body. This may eventually put a strain on them. If we do not use the extra protein for energy, the body will store it as fat.

ACTIVITY

1 Name two groups of people who need extra protein in their diet.
2 Give one reason why they need extra protein.
3 List four symptoms that you might expect to see in a child who is not getting enough protein in their diet.

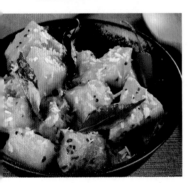

A vegan dish – pumpkin curry

PRACTICAL ACTIVITY

Make two main course vegan dishes and carry out a tasting panel to assess them for flavour, texture and acceptability for children.

Carry out a nutritional analysis of the recipes and comment on the protein content.

ACTIVITY

Match the key words below to their correct definitions.

Essential amino acids	Units that make up protein molecules
Low biological value	A protein food that does contain all the essential amino acids
Amino acids	A protein food that does not contain all the essential amino acids
High biological value	Must be provided ready-made by protein foods

ASSESSMENT FOR LEARNING

Read the case study below and answer the questions at the end.

Dan and Sonia are aged 27 and 26 years respectively. They have two children, Molly (four years old) and Amber (two years old). Sonia is expecting their third child.

Dan and Sonia want the whole family to have a vegan diet, which means that they will not eat any animal foods (meat, fish and poultry) or any animal food products (milk, butter, eggs, cheese, cream or yogurt). They will only eat plant foods, including vegetables, fruits, cereals, nuts, seeds and beans and bean products such as soya milk.

Sonia plans to breastfeed the new baby when it is born, as she did for the two girls.

Dan and Sonia want to make sure that their diet is good enough for the girls and the new baby to grow well and for the whole family to stay healthy.

1 What advice would you give to Dan and Sonia about their diet to help them understand how they can make sure that they have enough protein and energy?
2 Suggest a breakfast, lunch and evening meal that they and the children might like to eat.

1.2 FATS

WHAT ARE FATS?

Fat is a macronutrient. It can either be solid at room temperature or liquid at room temperature. Liquid fat is called oil. When a fat is heated it melts and becomes oil. When oil is chilled it solidifies (hardens) and becomes a fat.

The chemical name for a fat molecule is a triglyceride. Triglycerides are made of one part glycerol and three parts fatty acids. Fatty acids can be either saturated (full up) or unsaturated (not full up) with the element hydrogen. They look like this:

Saturated fatty acids	Unsaturated fatty acids
These are full up with hydrogen atoms and cannot take any more.	These are not full up with hydrogen atoms – they could take more by breaking the double bonds in the molecules and adding hydrogen.
Solid fats are mostly made of saturated fatty acids – butter, lard, suet, solid margarine, the fat on meat.	If there is one double bond it is called a monounsaturated fatty acid. If there are two or more double bonds it is called a polyunsaturated fatty acid. Liquid oils are mostly made of unsaturated fatty acids – sunflower oil, olive oil, rapeseed oil, corn oil, nut oil.

Hydrogenated fat

It is possible to make a solid fat, like margarine, from liquid oil by adding hydrogen under special conditions in a factory. The process is called hydrogenation.

Why does the body need fat?

Fat is the main store of energy in the body. It is stored in special cells under the skin called adipose tissue. This tissue insulates the body to stop it losing heat and protects the bones against physical damage by providing them with padding. Fat also gives us fat-soluble vitamins A, D, E and K (see page 54) and it has a very important job in forming cell walls throughout the body.

Which foods give us fat (sources of fat)?

Some fats and oils are visible (they are easy to see), such as the fat on cuts of meat, solid fats such as butter, lard and suet, margarine and low fat spreads and liquid oils (like the ones described above). Vitamins A and D are also added by law to margarine to make it have a similar nutritional value to butter.

Some fats and oils are invisible (they form part of the food and cannot be seen on their own), such as the fats and oils in avocados, oily fish (tuna, sardines, mackerel), cakes, pastries, biscuits, burgers and other meat products, chips, potato crisps, sausages, cheese, egg yolk, cream, fried foods, some ready-made meals, nuts, chocolate and ice cream.

Some foods naturally contain little fat, such as fruits (except avocados), vegetables, cereals (rice, wheat) and white fish (cod, plaice, haddock).

If you are not sure about the amount of fat in a food, it is important to read the nutrition information on food labels. These show the amount of fat in 100g of the product (see page 69).

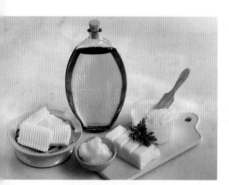
Visible fats and oils

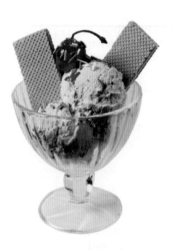
This food contains invisible fats

ACTIVITY

ACTIVITY

1 Give three reasons why our bodies need fat.
2 What is the name given to liquid fat?
3 What is the chemical name for a fat molecule?
4 Describe the difference between saturated fatty acids and unsaturated fatty acids.
5 Name three fats that are mostly made up of saturated fatty acids.
6 Name three oils that are mostly made up of unsaturated fatty acids.
7 Name three foods other than solid fats or oils that give us fat.
8 Name three foods that contain invisible fat (fat that we cannot see).
9 Name three foods that contain little fat.

How much fat do we need?

Fats should form a relatively small part of our meals everyday. The Eatwell plate (see page 67) shows how much we should have compared to other foods. Many people eat more than the recommended amount each day. This can increase their risk of developing diet-related health conditions such as heart disease.

There are various ways in which we can reduce the amount of fat we eat:

- Choose lean cuts of meat.
- When buying minced meat, check on the label for the fat content and try to buy minced meat that has no more than 5 per cent fat.
- Trim the fat from meat and poultry before cooking.
- Grill or oven bake foods such as meat, sausages and fish rather than fry them in fat or oil (because the fat will melt and drain away from the food).
- When shallow frying or stir frying food, if the food starts to become dry, add a little water rather than more oil to continue the cooking.
- Choose low or reduced fat versions of foods such as yogurt, cheese, milk, biscuits, low fat spreads.
- Reduce the amount of butter or margarine that you spread on bread.
- Instead of using mayonnaise in sandwiches or to mix salad ingredients, try using low fat versions of crème fraiche, salad dressing or fromage frais instead.
- Buy canned oily fish such as tuna and sardines in tomato sauce, water or brine instead of oil.
- Instead of adding butter or margarine to mashed potato, add wholegrain mustard.
- Instead of eating ice cream, try sorbet which has a low fat content.

What happens if we do not have enough fat?

Some fatty acids are essential for the correct growth and functioning of the body and must be obtained from food. If babies and young children do not have enough of these their normal growth will be affected. If we do not get enough energy from carbohydrate or fat in our food, we will use up our fat stores and become thinner. This will also mean that we may feel cold and will hurt our bones if we accidentally hit them.

ACTIVITY

The fat content of food is greatly increased if certain cooking methods or other ingredients are added to them. The chart below shows the difference in fat content of two naturally low fat foods when they are prepared and cooked in different ways.

Potatoes		Cod (a white fish)	
Preparation and cooking method	Amount of fat in 100g	Preparation and cooking method	Amount of fat in 100g
Boiled in water	0.3g	Steamed	0.9g
Boiled and mashed with butter	4.3g	Grilled	1.3g
Roasted in oil	4.5g	Cod in parsley sauce, boiled	2.8g
Made into chips and fried in oil	9.5g	Cod fish fingers fried in oil	14.1g
Potato crisps (sliced thinly and fried in oil)	37.6g	Dipped in batter and fried in oil	15.4g

1 Why do potato crisps have so much more fat in them than roasted potatoes?
2 Why does grilled fish have a lower fat content than fish fried in oil?

It is possible to buy low fat versions of various foods. The chart below shows the difference in the amount of fat in some examples of these.

Name of food	Amount of fat in 100g of the standard food	Amount of fat in 100g of a low fat version of the food
Cheddar cheese	34.4g	15.0g
Cottage cheese	3.9g	1.4g
Fromage frais	7.1g	0.2g
Soft (cream) cheese	31g	5g
Plain yogurt	3g	0.8g
Margarine spread	73.4g	40.5g
Canned sardines	14.1g (canned in oil)	9.6g (canned in brine)
Beef burgers (grilled)	24.4g	9.5g
Pork sausages (raw)	27.3g	10.6g

PRACTICAL ACTIVITY

Make your own low fat oven chips/potato wedges

Wash four large potatoes (do not peel them) and cut them into large chips (large chips have a small surface area compared to thin chips so they take up less oil).

Put 2 tablespoons of vegetable or olive oil into a bowl and add a little freshly ground black pepper and a teaspoon of Cajun spices (optional). Mix well.

Add the chips and stir well to coat them. Spread them on to a shallow roasting tin and bake in the oven (Gas 5/190°C) for 25 to 30 minutes until crispy and golden. Stir them half way through the cooking time.

What happens if we have too much fat?

Fat provides the body with a concentrated source of energy (over twice the amount that carbohydrate provides). If we eat too much fat and do not use up the energy will eaten, the body will store the excess energy in the adipose tissue, and we will gain weight. The extra fat may also build up in the liver and cause health problems.

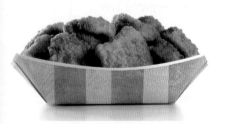

Processed foods, such as chicken nuggets, contain trans fats

ASSESSMENT FOR LEARNING

When you have worked through the rest of Topic 1.2, read the case study below and answer the questions at the end.

Simon is 42 years old and works in an office where he sits at a desk all day. In his free time he watches a lot of TV and uses a computer. He drives a car to and from work and rarely takes any exercise. His favourite foods are takeaway curries, fish and chips and pizzas, and he likes to eat crisps as a snack food. Simon was recently unwell with chest pains and his doctor has told him that this is a warning sign that he is developing heart disease. Simon is worried and wants to do something to prevent this from becoming worse.

1 What advice would you give Simon about his diet and lifestyle to help him improve his health?
2 Simon likes to cook. Suggest some menus he could follow and advise him on healthy ways he could cook his food.

Eating foods that are high in saturated fat can raise blood cholesterol levels, which increases the chances of developing heart disease (see page 74). There is also concern about the amount of hydrogenated fats that people eat.

Hydrogenated fats and oils are used in many processed and 'fast foods'. It has been discovered that the hydrogenation process can alter some of the fatty acids so that they turn into trans fats. The body is not able to use trans fats and health professionals think that they cause damage to some of the body's cells, which may lead to a variety of health problems including heart disease, some forms of cancer, diabetes, obesity and problems with the bones. Like saturated fats, trans fats can raise blood cholesterol levels.

PRACTICAL ACTIVITY

Plan and make two reduced fat versions of the types of meals Simon would enjoy, such as a curry or pizza.

Carry out a nutritional analysis of the recipes and comment on the fat content of your reduced fat recipes compared to typical ready-made versions.

ACTIVITY

Put the correct word from the list below into each of the following definitions about fat.

monounsaturated	hydrogenation	polyunsaturated
saturated	unsaturated	triglyceride

The chemical name for a fat molecule is a _____ .

A fatty acid that cannot take up any more hydrogen is called a _____ fat.

A fatty acid that has space for more hydrogen because some of the carbon atoms are joined with double bonds is called an _____ fat.

A fatty acid with one double bond between two carbon atoms is called _____ .

A fatty acid with two or more double bonds between carbon atoms is called _____ .

The name of the process for turning liquid oils into solid fats is _____ .

ASSESSMENT FOR LEARNING

Read the statements below and on a piece of paper, put a tick ✓ against all the ones you can do. If you can tick them all, well done! Make sure you can remember them in case you are asked to repeat them.

I can...

☐ Describe what a fat is and what an oil is

☐ Name three foods that contain visible fat food and three that contain invisible fat

☐ Explain what happens if the body has too much fat

☐ Explain why the body needs fat

☐ Identify which cooking methods add fat to

☐ Identify ways of reducing the amount of fat in the diet.

1.3 CARBOHYDRATES

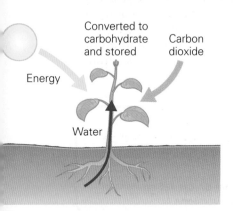

Energy — Converted to carbohydrate and stored — Carbon dioxide

Water

Photosynthesis

WHAT ARE CARBOHYDRATES?

Carbohydrate is a macronutrient. Carbohydrates are made by green plants during a process called photosynthesis. The plants use energy from sunlight to turn water (from the soil) and carbon dioxide gas (from the air) into carbohydrate, which they store in their roots, stems, fruits and leaves.

The energy is 'trapped' in the carbohydrate so when we eat it, the energy is released in our bodies. This means that plant foods are the most important sources of carbohydrate. There are two main types:

- sugars
- complex carbohydrates.

Sugars

Sugars are the simple units (molecules) from which all carbohydrates are made. There are two groups of sugars with different types in each.

Sugar group	Names of individual sugars	Foods which supply them
Simple sugars Chemical name: monosaccharides	Fructose	Fruits, plant juices, honey
	Glucose	Vegetables, fruits (especially when ripe), sugar used in cooking
	Galactose	Milk
Double sugars Chemical name: disaccharides	Sucrose Made from: 1 unit of glucose + 1 unit of fructose fruits and vegetables	Sugar cane and sugar beet (made into caster sugar, granulated sugar, brown sugar, etc.), also found in some
	Lactose Made from: 1 unit of glucose + 1 unit of galactose	Milk and some milk products such as yogurt
	Maltose Made from: 1 unit of glucose + 1 unit of glucose	Cereal plants such as barley, and added to products such as malted biscuits, malted milk drinks

Complex carbohydrates

Complex carbohydrates are made up of long 'chains' (molecules) of glucose units all joined together in different ways. There are five main groups of complex carbohydrates, which are also known as polysaccharides. Polysaccharide means 'poly' = many + 'saccharides' = sugars

Polysaccharide name	What it is and what it does	Foods which are good sources
Starch	• The main energy store for plants • Broken down during digestion to glucose units and used for energy in the body	• Root vegetables (e.g. carrots, parsnips), potatoes, yams, plantains, bananas, cereals (rice, wheat, millet, oats), cereal products (e.g. bread, pasta, pastries, biscuits, breakfast cereals), lentils, beans, seeds
Dietary fibre Chemical name: non-starch polysaccharides (NSP)	• The parts of a plant that give it strength and structure • Includes cellulose and gums • Cannot be digested by the body • Helps the body to get rid of solid waste products (faeces)	• Whole grain cereal foods (e.g. whole wheat, brown rice, oats), whole grain cereal products (e.g. bread, pasta, breakfast cereals, wheat and oat bran), seeds, beans, lentils, fruits and vegetables (especially leaves and stems)
Pectin	• Makes a gel in products such as jam so that the jam sets • Cannot be digested by the body • Helps the body to get rid of solid waste products (faeces)	• Some fruits (e.g. plums, apricots, damsons, apples)
Dextrin	• Formed during the baking and toasting of starchy products • Broken down during digestion to glucose units and used for energy in the body	• Toasted bread, the crust on cakes, bread, pastries
Glycogen	• Formed in the body in the liver from the digestion of carbohydrates • Stored in the liver and muscles as a supply of energy	• Made in the body

Why does the body need carbohydrates?

Carbohydrate is the main source of energy for the body. Every function of the body – movement, digestion of food, growth – needs a constant supply of energy to make it happen. So we need to have carbohydrate in our diet every day.

ACTIVITY

1 Give one reason why our bodies need carbohydrate.
2 Complete the sentence: 'Plant foods are the main source of carbohydrate and there are two types – these are sugars and _____ _____.'
3 What are monosaccharides? Give one example.
4 What are disaccharides? Give one example.
5 Name two foods that are good sources of simple sugars.
6 Name two foods that are good sources of double sugars.
7 What are polysaccharides?
8 Name two polysaccharides.
9 List three foods that are good sources of starch.
10 List three foods that are good sources of fibre.

ACTIVITY

Here is the ingredients list from a food label. Some food manufacturers use the chemical names for sugars and complex carbohydrates in their products.

> Ingredients:
> Sucrose, porridge oats, dextrose, wheat flakes, ground rice, dried apricots, soya beans, fructose, corn syrup, partially hydrogenated groundnut oil, milk powder, hazelnuts, honey, malt, modified starch, flavouring.

1 Identify the names of the sugars and the ingredients that contain complex carbohydrates that are in this product.
2 What type of a food product do you think it is?

How much carbohydrate do we need?

Complex carbohydrates should form the main part of our meals every day and should supply most of our energy. The Eatwell plate (see page 67) shows how much we should have compared to other foods.

What happens if we do not have enough carbohydrate?

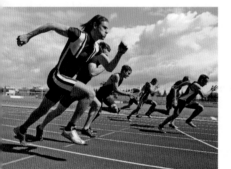

The body must have a constant supply of energy. It can also get energy from fat and protein foods, but prefers to use carbohydrate. If we do not eat enough carbohydrate, our bodies will use fat from our food intake and body stores, and we will lose weight. If there is still not enough from these sources, protein from the muscles will be broken down and converted to energy, but this is not good for the body and will weaken it.

In areas of the world where there are long-term food shortages and people suffer from famine, it is a common sight to see very thin people with little or no muscle on their bodies.

People who are training to take part in sports activities have to make sure that they have enough glycogen stored in their liver and muscles before they exercise. If they do not have enough, their muscles will run out of energy, they will start breaking down fat for energy (which is a much slower process) and will suffer from severe fatigue (tiredness) which is known as 'hitting the wall'. To prevent this, athletes must make sure they load their body with carbohydrate in the days before a sporting event so that their liver and muscle glycogen stores are full.

What happens if we have too much carbohydrate?

If we eat too much carbohydrate and do not use up the energy we have eaten, the body will store the excess energy from the carbohydrate as fat in special tissue called adipose tissue under the skin.

ACTIVITY

1 Why does someone who works as a builder need more carbohydrate than someone who works in an office?
2 If someone has put on a lot of weight, what should they do to try and lose weight?

ACTIVITY

Complete the words below.
1 The production of carbohydrates by green plants is called _ _ o _ o _ y _ t _ e _ i _.
2 Simple sugar units are called _ o _ o _ a _ _ h _ r _ d _ s.
3 Double sugars are called _ _ s a _ _ h _ r _ d _ s and are made from two _ o _ o _ a _ _ h _ r _ d _ s joined together.
4 Complex carbohydrates are made from many glucose units joined together and are called _ o l _ s a _ _ h _ r _ d _ s.

PRACTICAL ACTIVITY

Plan and make two recipes (e.g. main meals, snacks, breakfast items) that would help the teenagers in the Assessment for learning case study load their bodies with glycogen.

Carry out a nutritional analysis of the recipes and comment on the carbohydrate content.

ASSESSMENT FOR LEARNING

Read the case study below and answer the questions at the end.

A group of teenagers are planning to take part in a half marathon to raise money for a local charity. As part of their training, they are going to take advice about what to eat to make sure that they have enough glycogen stored in their liver and muscles.

1 What advice would you give them about loading their bodies with carbohydrate before the marathon?
2 Suggest some meals they could eat.

1.4 WATER SOLUBLE VITAMINS

WHAT ARE VITAMINS?

Vitamins are micronutrients. They are natural substances found in foods that do different jobs in the body. Each vitamin is given a letter to identify it (e.g. vitamin C), but they also have chemical names. It is useful to know these because they are often used on food labels and in books and other sources of information.

Water soluble vitamins

These vitamins dissolve in water. They include the vitamin B group (there is more than one vitamin B) and vitamin C.

Vitamin B group

Scientists originally thought there was only one vitamin in this group, but then discovered that there were several more that had similar jobs in the body. So they were all grouped together and are sometimes known as the 'vitamin B complex'.

This topic tells you:

• the chemical names of each vitamin in the vitamin B complex
• why the body needs these vitamins
• the foods which give us these vitamins
• what happens if we do not have enough (a deficiency) of these vitamins
• what happens to these vitamins when foods are processed and cooked.

> ### ACTIVITY
>
> Using the information in this topic, find out the following information about each of the B vitamins (B1, B2, B3, B5, B6, B9 and B12):
> - the chemical name of the vitamin
> - two functions it has in the body
> - two sources of the vitamin
> - one deficiency caused by a lack of it.

Vitamin B_1 (Thiamin)

Function (its job in the body):

- It helps to release enery from carbohydrates
- It helps the body to grow
- It helps the nerves to work properly.

Sources (the foods it is found in):

- It is not stored in the body, so a supply is needed every day
- Cereals such as wheat and rice (especially whole grain) and cereal products, wheatgerm (from the wheat seeds)
- Yeast and yeast extracts (Marmite)
- All types of meat (especially pork, bacon, ham, liver, kidney, heart)
- Eggs, fish roe (eggs)
- Milk and dairy foods
- Seeds, nuts, beans.

Deficiency (what happens if we do not have enough):

- The body will develop a disease called beri-beri. There are two types:
  - Wet beri beri
  - Dry beri beri
- Beri beri often causes muscle wastage. It is usually only seen in communities where there is little to eat and where they eat a lot of polished white rice (where the outside layers of the rice have been removed) and not much else. It is also sometimes seen in people who are addicted to alcohol.

Effects of processing and cooking:

- Easily detroyed by heat when cooking
- Easily dissolves in water.

Vitamin B_2 (Riboflavin)

Function (its job in the body): helps to release energy from carbohydrates, fats and proteins.

Sources (the foods it is found in): the same as thiamin.

Deficiency (what happens if we do not have enough): low intakes can lead to dryness and cracking of the skin around the mouth and nose, and a swollen tongue.

Effects of processing and cooking: damaged by exposure to sunlight, such as milk left in a glass bottle on a doorstep after being delivered (although most milk is now sold in plastic containers and bought from shops).

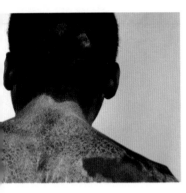

Pellagra

Vitamin B₃ (Niacin)

Function (its job in the body):

- It helps to release energy from food
- It can be used to lower the levels of fat in the blood.

Sources (the foods it is found in):

- The same as thiamin and riboflavin
- Also, niacin can be made in the body from an amino acid (see page 39) called tryptophan.

Deficiency (what happens if we do not have enough):

- The body will develop a disease called pellagra (the word comes from two Italian words: 'pelle' meaning skins and 'agro' meaning sour). The symptoms of pellagra are known as the 'three Ds':
  - Diarrhoea
  - Dermatitis (roughened, sore skin)
  - Dementia (confusion, memory loss, unable to speak properly).

Vitamin B₅ (Pantothenic acid)

Function (its job in the body): helps to release energy from food.

Sources (the foods it is found in): a wide range of foods.

Deficiency (what happens if we do not have enough): A deficiency is rare.

Vitamin B₆ (Pyridoxine)

Function (its job in the body): helps the body to use protein, fat and carbohydrate for different jobs.

Sources (the foods it is found in): found in small amounts in a wide range of foods.

Deficiency (what happens if we do not have enough): can lead to headaches, general aching and weakness, anaemia (a problem with the cells in the blood) and skin problems.

Effects of processing and cooking: can be destroyed during cooking.

Vitamin B₉ (Folate)

Folate is the natural form of the vitamin. There is also a man-made form called folic acid.

Function (its job in the body):

- It helps the body to use protein
- It has a very important job to make a special material called DNA in the body cells, when they divide to produce more cells, especially the cells in the bone marrow (which produce red blood cells) and the cells that line the digestive system.

Sources (the foods it is found in):

- Green and leafy vegetables – spinach and green cabbage
- Liver
- Potatoes
- Fruits – oranges and berries
- Asparagus, okra
- Beans and sees
- Wholegrain cereals
- Nuts
- Folic acid is also added to breakfast cereals.

Deficiency (what happens if we do not have enough):

- A deficiency can lead to cells in the digestive system not dividing properly, so other nutrients are not absorbed. This can lead to loss of appetite, nausea (feeling sick), diarrhoea and soreness in the mouth
- A deficiency can also lead to cells in the bone marrow not dividing properly which will lead to the red blood cells becoming very large and not being able to deliver enough oxygen around the body. This is called megaloblastic anaemia ('mega' meaning big, 'blastic' meaning cells, 'anaemia' meaning not enough active red blood cells in the blood)
- In the very first stages of pregnancy large numbers of cells develop and divide to produce all the different parts of the body. Pregnant women need about five times more folate than normal. One of the vital stages of pregnancy is the development of the spinal cord and backbone. If a woman does not have enough folate, her baby may develop a deformity in the spine called spina bifida. It is important that women have enough folate in their diet before they conceive a baby and in the first few months of pregnancy to avoid this. Folic acid supplements are given to make sure that such women have enough in their diet.

Effects of processing and cooking:

- Folate is less sensitive to heat than other B vitamins but it will be destroyed if food is reheated or kept hot for a while
- Folic acid is more stable when cooking and in the digestive system, so is more likely to be absorbed into the body

Vitamin B$_{12}$ (Cobalamin)

Function (its job in the body):

- It is needed to form a protective coating around nerve cells to make them work properly
- It is important for the correct production of new cells.

Sources (the foods it is found in):

- It can be stored in the liver
- It is only found in foods from animals (meat, milk, dairy products and liver), so vegans (people who do not eat any animal products) need to make sure they take a supplement.

Deficiency (what happens if we do not have enough):

- A deficiency will prevent the nerves from working properly and will lead to paralysis, memory loss and confusion
- A type of anaemia called pernicious anaemia can occur in people who have had certain medical conditions that stop the vitamin B12 from being absorbed.

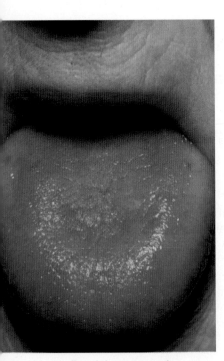

Pernicious anaemia

Vitamin C

This topic tells you:

- the chemical name for vitamin C
- why the body needs vitamin C
- the foods which give us vitamin C
- what happens if we do not have enough (a deficiency) vitamin C
- what happens to vitamin C when foods are processed and cooked
- how to conserve vitamin C in foods when you are preparing and cooking them.

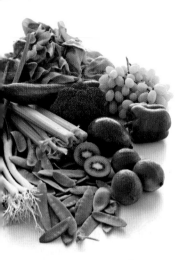

Sources of vitamin C

ACTIVITY

Use the following information to answer these questions:

1 What is the chemical name of vitamin C?
2 Describe two functions of vitamin C in the body.
3 Name three sources of vitamin C.
4 Identify the deficiency disease caused by a lack of vitamin C and describe two of the symptoms.
5 Suggest three ways of conserving vitamin C when preparing and cooking vegetables.

ACTIVITY

1 Why do raw foods usually have higher vitamin levels than cooked foods?
2 Why do fruits and vegetables that have just been picked usually have the highest vitamin levels?

Vitamin C (Ascorbic acid)

Function (its job in the body):

- It is needed to enable the body to absorb iron from the food we eat
- It is needed for the production of a protein in the body called collagen
- Collagen is the protein in connective tissue which is the substance that binds the body cells together
- It is also an antioxidant. Antioxidants help to protect the body from polluting chemicals that get into the body – from the air, water or in food.

Sources (the foods it is found in):

- Fruits and vegetables, especially blackcurrants, citrus fruits, green peppers, kiwi fruit, green, leafy vegetables (not lettuce), Brussels sprouts, broccoli, bean sprouts, peas, potatoes (we eat a lot of potatoes so they give us an important amount)
- There is a small amount in liver and fresh milk.

Deficiency (what happens if we do not have enough):

- A deficiency is rare but is occasionally seen in older adults and some children who have very little fresh fruit and vegetables in their diet
- The body is able to store some vitamin C, but we cannot make it in our bodies and so need some every day in our diet
- If someone has a slight deficiency, anaemia develops because not enough iron is absorbed. The symptoms are tiredness and weakness
- A severe deficiency leads to the disease scurvy which has the following symptoms:

- tiredness and weakness
- bleeding gums
- anaemia
- poor wound healing and damage to bone and other tissues.

Effects of processing and cooking:

- Vitamin C is destroyed by heat and exposure to oxygen
- It dissolves very easily in water (water soluble).

To prevent this, it is important to prepare and cook fruits and vegetables in the following way:

- Buy them as fresh as possible (so they have the most vitamin C)
- Prepare them at the last minute before you need them to avoid long exposure to the air
- Cook them in as little water as possible (steaming is a better method), for as short a time as possible and serve them straightaway – do not keep them hot for a while before serving
- Use the water they were cooked in for making gravy or soup.

1.5 FAT SOLUBLE VITAMINS

WHAT ARE FAT SOLUBLE VITAMINS?

There are four vitamins in this group. They are vitamins A, D, E and K. They dissolve in fat.

This topic tells you:

- the chemical names of each fat soluble vitamin
- why the body needs these vitamins
- the foods which give us these vitamins
- what happens if we do not have enough (a deficiency) of these vitamins
- what happens to these vitamins when foods are processed and cooked.

ACTIVITY

Use the following information to answer these questions.

1 Describe two functions of vitamin A in the body.
2 Name two sources of vitamin A from animal foods and two sources from plant foods.
3 Identify one deficiency disease caused by lack of vitamin A.
4 Describe two functions of vitamin D in the body.
5 Name two foods that provide us with vitamin D.
6 Apart from food, how else do we get vitamin D?
7 What happens to our bodies if we do not get enough vitamin D?
8 Name the deficiency disease caused by lack of vitamin D.

RESEARCH ACTIVITY

1 Find out why vitamins A and D are added to margarine by law.
2 A lot of poor children who lived in cities in the UK during the early part of the twentieth century developed rickets. Why do you think this was, and why is it rare to see it now?

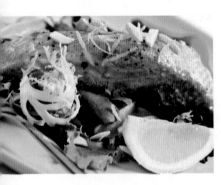

Lettuce is a source of vitamin E; salmon is a source of vitamins A and D

Vitamin A (Retinol in animal food sources or beta carotene in plant food sources)

Function (its job in the body):
- It helps the body grow and develop
- It keeps the lining of the throat, the digestive system and the lungs moist and free from infection
- It keeps the skin healthy
- It makes a substance called visual purple, in the retina at the back of the eye so we can see well enough in dim light to stop us bumping into things
- It is an antioxidant so it helps stop substances that get into the body from the air, water and elsewhere from damaging it.

Vitamin A is found in foods in two different forms:
- as retinol in animal foods, e.g. milk, cheese, butter, oily fish (e.g. tuna, herrings, mackerel, sardines), liver and liver products e.g. pate
- as beta carotene in plant foods, e.g. carrots, oranges, red peppers, saffron, dark green leafy vegetables, tomatoes, palm fruit, apricots, margarine (added by law, a process called fortification)

Beta carotene is changed to retinol in the body.

Deficiency (what happens if we do not have enough):
- Children do not grow properly
- It becomes difficult for the body to fight infection
- The person will not be able to see in dim light – this is called night blindness
- This will eventually lead to blindness – a condition known as keratomalacia (very common in poor countries)
- Too much vitamin A is poisonous to the body. People should be careful when they take vitamin supplements and should only do so on the advice of their doctor.

Vitamin A is not affected by most cooking processes.

Vitamin D (Cholecalciferol)

This is how you say it: Co-lee-cal-siff-er-ol.

Function (its job in the body):
- Vitamin D controls the amount of calcium that is absorbed from food in the body
- It also helps us to develop strong bones and teeth by making sure that they take up plenty of minerals such as calcium and phosphorus. It is important that the bones reach their 'peak bone mass' during childhood, adolescence and early adulthood so that they are their strongest and will last a long time without becoming weak.

Sources (the food it is found in):
- A few foods contain some vitamin D – liver, oily fish, butter, cheese, milk and eggs and it is added by law to margarine
- Most of our vitamin D comes from exposure of the skin to sunlight. When the rays of the sun reach the skin, a chemical reaction takes place under the skin to form vitamin D, which is then stored in the liver.

Deficiency (what happens if we do not have enough):
- A deficiency of vitamin D means that not enough calcium is absorbed from food, and the bones and teeth do not become strong enough
- The weak bones bend under the weight of the body and become deformed. In children this disease is called rickets and if it happens in adults it is called osteomalacia (means 'bad' bones)
- Osteomalacia is not the same as osteoporosis, which is a natural process where the bones become weaker as people get older.

Vitamin D is not affected by normal cooking processes.

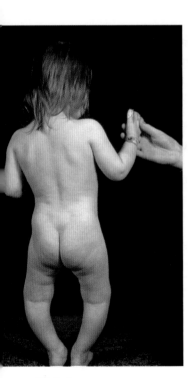
Rickets

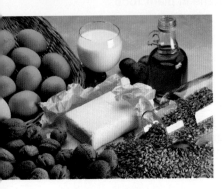

Dairy products provide vitamins A and D; oil and seeds provide vitamin E; eggs provide vitamin D; nuts provide calcium

Vitamin E (Tocopherol)

This is how you say it: Tock-off-er-ol.

Function (its job in the body):
- Vitamin E is an antioxidant so it helps stop substances that get into the body from the air, water and elsewhere from damaging it
- It is needed to make sure that the cell walls in the body stay healthy
- It is thought to reduce the risk of people developing some types of cancers and heart disease.

Sources (the food it is found in): vegetable oils, lettuce, grasses, peanuts, seeds and wheatgerm oil.

A deficiency of vitamin E is rare.

Vitamin E is not affected by normal cooking processes.

Vitamin K

Function (its job in the body): helps the blood to clot. This means that when we bleed following an injury, the blood will thicken and 'clot' at the place where the injury took place in order to allow it to be repaired and to stop us from losing too much blood.

Sources (the food it is found in):
- Vitamin K is found in plant and animal foods especially leafy vegetables, cheese, liver, asparagus, coffee, bacon and green tea
- It is also made by bacteria that live naturally in our intestines.

Deficiency (what happens if we do not have enough):
- Deficiency is very rare in adults, but is sometimes seen in newborn babies
- To prevent this, a dose of vitamin K is normally given to babies straight after birth, either by mouth or an injection.

Vitamin K is not affected by normal cooking processes.

ACTIVITY

Match each word with its correct definition by drawing arrows between each of the lists.

Deficiency disease	A substance that dissolves in water
Water soluble	A group of vitamins that have similar jobs in the body
Fat soluble	A food that gives you a nutrient
Vitamin complex	A substance that dissolves in fats or oils
Source	An illness or condition in the body caused by not having enough of a nutrient in the diet

PRACTICAL ACTIVITY

Cook one or two of the meals (main course and dessert) that you plan in the Assessment for learning activity, and set up a tasting panel to assess the suitability of the meals for elderly people.

Carry out a nutritional analysis of the recipes and comment on the vitamin content (fat and water soluble) of your recipes. How would you improve or conserve the vitamin content?

ASSESSMENT FOR LEARNING

Read the case study below and answer the questions at the end.

A group of people are starting a lunch club for some elderly people who mostly live alone. Some of the elderly people do not have very healthy diets because they find it difficult to cook for themselves.

The organisers of the club want to make sure that the elderly guests get as many vitamins from the food as possible to help keep them healthy, so they are planning their menus carefully. They want the elderly guests to have a variety of tasty meals to encourage them to eat and enjoy their food as well as the company of other guests.

There will be 30 elderly guests to cater for each week.

1 How can the people who are cooking the food avoid losing vitamins (especially the water soluble vitamins) during preparation, cooking and serving?
2 Plan some tasty two-course meals that could be served to the elderly guests that will contain plenty of vitamins.

1.6 MINERALS AND TRACE ELEMENTS

WHAT ARE MINERALS AND TRACE ELEMENTS?

Minerals and trace elements are micronutrients. They are chemical elements that do not contain carbon and are needed by the body for a variety of jobs.

Minerals are needed by adults in quantities of between 1mg and 100mg per day and they include calcium, iron, magnesium, phosphorus, potassium, sodium chromium, copper, manganese, selenium, sulphur and zinc.

Trace elements are needed by adults in quantities of less than 1mg a day (which is very small) and they include fluoride, iodine, cobalt, molybdenum and silicon.

All of the minerals and trace elements are essential for the body, but in this topic we are going to study just five of them: calcium, iron, sodium, fluoride and iodine.

This topic tells you:
- why the body needs these minerals and trace elements
- the foods which give us these minerals and trace elements
- what happens if we do not have enough (a deficiency) of these minerals and trace elements
- what happens to these minerals and trace elements when foods are processed and cooked.

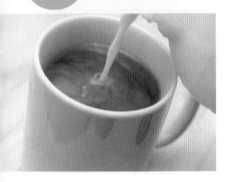

Tea contains fluoride; milk is a source of calcium and iodine

Calcium

Function (its job in the body):

- It is needed for normal growth in children
- It is the main mineral in bones and teeth and gives them strength and hardness
- It is needed to help the blood to clot after an injury
- It is needed to help the nerves and muscles work properly.

Sources (the foods it is found in):

- Vitamin D is needed to help the body absorb calcium from food
- It is found in milk and dairy products such as cheese and yogurt
- It is found in plant foods such as wholegrain cereals, seeds, nuts, green leafy vegetables and lentils
- Calcium is added to some foods to enrich them – white bread has calcium added by law and some products such as milk, soya milk, fruit juices and yogurt have extra calcium added to them.

Deficiency (what happens if we do not have enough):

- As we grow, our bones gradually get bigger and stronger as calcium and other minerals are laid down in them
- Physical, load-bearing exercise such as running, jumping and walking stimulates the bones to take up minerals, so it is essential for children and teenagers to be physically active to help this process
- It is essential that we have enough calcium in our diets to allow the bones to reach their peak bone mass (this is when they are hardest and have the most minerals in them and is particularly important during adolescence)
- If the bones do not reach peak bone mass, they gradually become weaker as we grow older and will be more likely to break
- If a pregnant woman does not have enough calcium in her diet, calcium will be removed from her bones to enable the bones of the unborn baby to grow. This will weaken the woman's bones and teeth
- If there is not enough calcium in the blood, the blood will not clot properly after an injury and the nerves and muscles will not work properly, leading to a condition called 'tetany' in which the muscles become rigid and will not relax.

Calcium is not affected by normal cooking processes.

Iron

Function (its job in the body): iron is needed to make a red-coloured protein called haemoglobin in red blood cells (which is why blood is red), which take oxygen around the body.

Sources (the foods it is found in):

- Vitamin C is needed to help the body absorb iron from food
- Good sources of iron include red meat, liver, kidney, dried apricots, lentils, corned beef, curry spices, cocoa and plain chocolate. There is also some iron in egg yolk
- Bread and many breakfast cereals are fortified with iron
- Green leafy vegetables, e.g. spinach, contain some iron but not all of it may be available to the body.

Deficiency (what happens if we do not have enough):

- Newborn babies have a supply of iron that lasts about three months (milk is a poor source of iron) until the baby starts to be weaned on to solid foods
- Adolescent girls and women must make sure they have enough iron in their diet to cope with the loss of iron during their periods

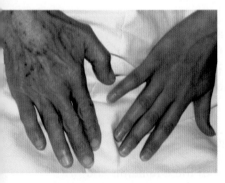

Iron-deficiency anaemia: comparing an anaemic hand with a healthy hand

- Pregnant women must have enough iron in their diet to supply their own increased blood volume and the baby's store
- A deficiency of iron leads to low iron stores in the body and eventually to iron deficiency anaemia
- Symptoms of anaemia include:
  – tiredness, weakness, lack of energy
  – a pale complexion, pale inner eyelids
  – weak and split fingernails.

Effects of processing and cooking:

- Iron is not affected by normal cooking processes
- It is a good idea to eat foods rich in vitamin C with iron-rich foods to help the absorption of iron.

Sodium

Function (its job in the body):

- Sodium is needed to control the amount of water in the body
- It is also needed to help the body use energy and to control the nerves and muscles.

Sources (the foods it is found in):

- Salt is sodium chloride
- Most raw foods contain very small amounts of sodium chloride (salt)
- During the processing, preparation, preservation and serving of many foods salt is added – snack foods (crisps, roasted salted nuts) ready meals and instant foods such as dried soups and pasta pot meals, takeaway foods, cheese, yeast extract, canned fish, smoked flavour foods such as bacon, ham and fish
- Sodium is also found in sodium bicarbonate which is used as a raising agent in baked foods such as cakes and biscuits
- Sodium is also found in a food additive called monosodium glutamate which is used to increase the flavour in many takeaway foods and ready meals.

Deficiency (what happens if we do not have enough):

- A deficiency of sodium will cause muscle cramps and is sometimes seen in people who work or take part in sports in very hot conditions because they lose sodium in their sweat
- The body can also lose too much sodium if someone has sickness and diarrhoea
- Many people have too much salt in their diet (see page 70)
- If you have too much salt, you may develop high blood pressure which puts a strain on the heart and other parts of the body
- Too much salt can also damage the kidneys, especially in babies and young children.

Sodium is not affected by normal cooking methods.

Fluoride

Function (its job in the body): to help strengthen the bones and the enamel part of the teeth.

Sources (the foods it is found in): in sea water fish, tea and naturally in some water supplies.

Deficiency (what happens if we do not have enough): the teeth may be more likely to develop cavities (holes) if they are not cared for properly.

Fluoride is not affected by normal cooking processes.

ASSESSMENT FOR LEARNING

Look at the statements below for each mineral and trace element. Put a tick ✓ against all the ones you can do. If you can tick them all, well done! Make sure you can remember them in case you are asked to repeat them.

Calcium: I can...

☐ Describe what peak bone mass is

☐ Explain why the body needs calcium

☐ Name three foods that are good sources of calcium

☐ Identify two stages in people's lives when having plenty of calcium is particularly important

☐ Explain what happens if the body does not have enough calcium

☐ Identify the vitamin that is needed to help us absorb calcium from food

Iron: I can...

☐ Describe why blood is red

☐ Explain why the body needs iron

☐ Name three foods that are good sources of iron

☐ Identify why it is particularly important for teenage girls and women to have enough iron

☐ Explain what happens if the body does not have enough iron

☐ Identify the vitamin that is needed to help us absorb iron from food

Sodium: I can...

☐ Describe which types of food contain sodium apart from those with added salt in them

☐ Explain why the body needs sodium

☐ Name three foods that are natural sources of sodium

☐ Identify three foods that have salt added to them when they are processed

☐ Explain what happens if the body does not have enough sodium

☐ Identify why it is not good for the body if we have too much salt in our diet

Fluoride: I can...

☐ Describe what can happen to teeth if they are not looked after properly

☐ Explain why the body needs fluoride

☐ Name two sources of fluoride

☐ Identify a cosmetic product that we use every day that has fluoride added to it

☐ Explain what happens if the body does not have enough fluoride

Iodine: I can...

☐ Describe where the thyroid gland is in the body

☐ Explain why the body needs iodine

☐ Name two foods that are good sources of iodine

☐ Identify why plant and dairy foods vary in the amount of iodine they contain

☐ Explain what happens if the body does not have enough iodine

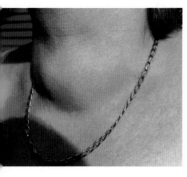

Goitre

Iodine

Function (its job in the body):

- It is needed to make thyroid hormones in the thyroid gland in the neck
- Thyroid hormones control the metabolic rate of the body – the rate at which chemical reactions take place inside the body.

Sources (the food it is found in):

- It is found in sea foods
- It is also found in milk and dairy foods and some plant foods depending on how rich in iodine the soil is in the area in which the cows or plants have grown.

Deficiency (what happens if we do not have enough):

- The person will feel tired, lethargic (does not want to do anything) and will gain weight
- The thyroid gland in the neck will swell up to form a goitre (this is how you say it: 'goy-ter').

Iodine is not affected by normal cooking processes.

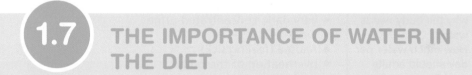

1.7 THE IMPORTANCE OF WATER IN THE DIET

WHY DOES THE BODY NEED WATER?

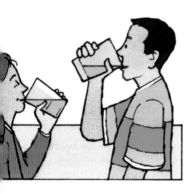

Water is not usually called a nutrient, but it is essential for life and the body will suffer and die within a few days if we do not have any water in our diet.

Our bodies are made up of about 60 per cent water. Water has many jobs in the body including:

- It is found in all cells and tissues.
- It is part of most chemical reactions in the body.
- It is found in all body fluids – including blood, saliva, digestive juices, sweat, urine and the fluid in joints such as the knee.
- It controls our body temperature of 37°C by taking heat out of the body when we sweat.
- It helps get rid of waste products from the body as urine (from the kidneys) and in faeces (from the digestive system).
- It keeps the linings of the digestive system, mucous membranes (inside the nose and mouth) and the lungs moist and healthy.
- It helps us absorb nutrients.
- It helps to keep the concentration of substances in the blood, such as dissolved minerals (known as electrolytes), at the right level.
- It helps to prevent the skin from drying out.

How much water should we drink?

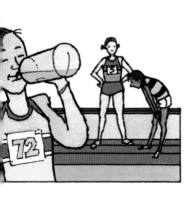

We get water from:

- the water we drink
- water that is naturally found in or added to foods.

Dietary guidelines recommend that adults should drink 1.75 to 2 litres of water per day (about six or seven average sized glasses), plus take in water from food to replace daily losses. This requirement will increase if we are in a hot climate and will also increase with physical activity and exercise.

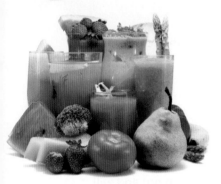

Foods that give us water

Which are the best sources of drinking water?

In the UK, drinking water from taps is safe to drink because the water has been treated to kill dangerous organisms such as bacteria and certain types of algae that could cause illness.

Which foods give us water?

Apart from drinking water on its own or in drinks such as fruits juices, milk and tea, we also get water from foods. Fruits and vegetables have the highest amounts of water, and the water is taken from the soil and into the plants by their roots as they grow. Foods such as cereal grains, meat and fish have less water in them and do not contribute much to our water intake.

What happens if we do not have enough water?

Most people do not drink enough water. If we do not have enough, the 'thirst centre' in our brain (called the hypothalamus) makes us feel thirsty to make us drink some water.

A lack of water in the body is called dehydration. It leads to a variety of symptoms including:

- headache
- very dark, concentrated urine
- weakness
- nausea (feeling sick)
- overheating of the body
- confusion
- sunken eyes
- changes in blood pressure
- rapid heart beat
- loose, wrinkled skin.

If the body loses 20 per cent of its water, this will result in death. Dehydration is particularly dangerous for babies and young children, elderly people and patients with kidney diseases.

What happens if we have too much water?

Having too much water is called water intoxication. If you drink too much water, eventually the kidneys will not be able to work fast enough to remove it from the body, so the blood becomes too diluted. This can cause the brain to swell, headaches, nausea, vomiting, muscle twitching, convulsions and even death.

ACTIVITY

1 Give four reasons why the body needs water.
2 How much water per day should adults drink?
3 Name two foods that have a high water content.
4 What is meant by dehydration?
5 Identify (list) four symptoms that can be caused by a lack of water.
6 Suggest two reasons for needing an increased daily intake of water.

RESEARCH ACTIVITY

1 How could you include more water in the diet of a child who is reluctant to drink it?
2 Why is it not a good idea to increase your daily liquid intake by drinking lots of sweet, carbonated (fizzy) drinks?
3 An athletics team are training to take part in a major games contest in southern Italy during the summer. They will be arriving at the venue a week before the games start in order to prepare themselves and get used to the climate. What precautions will they need to take to make sure that they do not become dehydrated?
4 Suggest some foods that they could eat to make sure they maintain their blood salt concentrations.

ASSESSMENT FOR LEARNING

Your school is trying to encourage pupils to drink more water. Design a poster that could be produced and displayed in the school.

The poster should tell pupils why they need to drink water and the symptoms of not drinking enough water.

1.8 THE IMPORTANCE OF FIBRE IN THE DIET

WHAT IS FIBRE?

To help you understand fibre, you need to remember what you have learned about carbohydrates. Can you remember what starch is and what polysaccharides are?

Fibre is the name given to a group of natural plant materials that our bodies cannot digest (break down). Fibre used to be called 'roughage', then it became 'dietary fibre' and then it was shortened to 'fibre'. The proper scientific name for fibre is non-starch polysaccharide (NSP). You may see this on food labels.

Fibre includes:

* cellulose: this is found in stems, leaves, leaf stalks, the outside layers of seeds and beans, and the peel on fruits and vegetables
* pectin: this is found in fruits such as plums, apples and blackcurrants and it is the substance that makes jam set.

Why does the body need fibre?

Fibre is needed by the body to help it get rid of solid waste matter (faeces). It does this by making the faeces bulky, soft and heavy so that they can move easily through the intestines and out of the body when we go to the toilet. This helps the intestines stay healthy and work properly

Fibre makes you feel full up after a meal so that you are less likely to eat more food between meals. It also helps to reduce the amount of cholesterol (see page 45) in the blood.

What happens if the body does not have enough fibre?

Too little fibre in the diet causes constipation. This is when people find it very difficult to get rid of faeces when they go to the toilet because the faeces are hard, small and dry. People with constipation often say they feel 'bloated', uncomfortable, irritable, tired and unwell. This is because the body wants to get rid of the waste products in faeces, which it cannot use and which could cause harm to the body. Because they are stuck inside, they cause these symptoms.

In some people who are often constipated, the faeces cause the lining of the intestines to become irritated and damaged. This could eventually lead to a disease called diverticular disease. The symptoms are pain and discomfort in the intestines caused by the development of small pouches in the lining of the intestines. These pouches become infected with bacteria and are very painful.

A low fibre intake can increase the risk of developing cancer in the intestines, especially in the bowel.

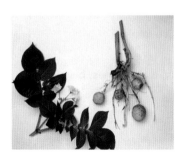

Plant materials contain fibre

How much fibre do we need?

We need some fibre in our diet every day. Current dietary guidelines recommend that adults should have a minimum of 18g a day, but the ideal amount for good health is 30g a day.

Children should have less because they are smaller, and it is recommended that for children under five years old, high fibre foods should be introduced to their diet gradually. If young children have too much fibre, their diet will be very bulky and they will feel full up before they have eaten enough food to give their bodies enough vitamins, minerals and energy.

A diet rich in fibre is usually low in fat and contains more starchy foods, fruit and vegetables.

We also need to drink plenty of water to help the fibre make the faeces soft and to take plenty of exercise to help the blood circulation reach the intestines so that they work properly

ACTIVITY

1 What is fibre?
2 Give three reasons why our bodies need fibre.
3 Identify (list) three health problems that can develop if a person does not get enough fibre.
4 What is the ideal amount of fibre that we should eat each day?
5 Identify (list) five foods that are good sources of fibre.
6 Identify (list) five foods that are poor sources of fibre.
7 Your friend is making spaghetti Bolognese using spaghetti made from white flour. How can the fibre content of the dish be increased?
8 Why are jacket potatoes a better source of fibre than mashed potatoes?

Which foods give us fibre?

Fibre is only found in foods which are from plants. Natural plant foods which have not been processed contain the most fibre.

The chart below shows which foods give us fibre.

Good sources of fibre	Poor sources of fibre
Wholemeal, granary or seeded bread	White bread
Wholegrain breakfast cereals, e.g. shredded wheat, bran flakes, weetabix, muesli, porridge oats	Breakfast cereals such as rice krispies, cornflakes, chocolate coated rice cereal, frosted cornflakes
Wholemeal pasta	Pasta made from white flour
Wholegrain (brown) rice	White (polished) rice
Wholemeal flour	White flour
Fresh fruits – especially with peel or skins	Smooth fruit juices and fruit juice drinks
Dried fruits	Sweets and chocolate
Vegetables – especially with peel or skins	Products made from white flour, e.g. pastries, biscuits, cakes
Nuts	
Seeds, linseeds, pumpkin seeds	
Beans, peas, lentils	

There are various ways in which we can increase the amount of fibre we eat each day, as the list below shows:

- Eat whole grain (wholemeal) breakfast cereals, bread, rice and pasta.
- Use wholemeal flour (either all wholemeal or half wholemeal and half white) for recipes such as cakes, scones, pastries, biscuits, bread, crumbles and sponge puddings.
- Add oat or wheat bran (available from supermarkets in the breakfast cereal section) to crumble toppings, cake, pastry and biscuit recipes.
- Add chopped fresh or dried fruits to your breakfast cereal.
- Add chopped dried fruits to cake, scone and biscuit recipes.
- Eat porridge for breakfast and add stewed fruit such as apples, plums and prunes.
- Eat plenty of fresh fruits, salads and vegetables and leave the skins and peel on where you can.
- Make delicious fruit smoothies with a blender, using a variety of fresh fruits.
- Eat dried fruits as snacks.
- Add peas, beans and lentils to stews, soups, curries – you can use dried, canned or frozen peas, beans and lentils.
- Add finely chopped vegetables to dishes such as Bolognese and curry.
- Make soups using a variety of vegetables – these can be blended or chunky.
- Add seeds to crumbles, breads, stews, soups, breakfast cereals, biscuit and cake mixtures.

The more natural (unprocessed) a plant food is, the more fibre it will contain. For example, wholegrain, unprocessed brown rice contains seven times more fibre than processed white rice!

ACTIVITY

Read the chart below, which shows the amount of fibre in different types of breakfast cereals. Then answer the questions below.

Types of breakfast cereal	Amount of fibre in a 30g serving
Sugar frosted cornflakes	0.36g
Chocolate coated rice cereal	0.33g
Crisp rice cereal	0.33g
Puffed wheat cereal	2.64g
Sugar coated puffed wheat cereal	1.44g
All bran	9.00g
Bran flakes	5.19g
Cornflakes	1.02g
Nut and honey cornflakes	0.48g
Fruit and fibre cereal	3.03g
Muesli	2.43g
Shredded wheat	3.03g

1 Which cereal has the most fibre?
2 Which cereal has the least fibre?
3 Which foods could be added to breakfast cereals to increase the amount of fibre?

RESEARCH ACTIVITY

1 Why is it important to eat plenty of fibre, drink plenty of water and take exercise in order to prevent constipation?
2 Elderly people or people who have been ill in bed for a while often have problems with constipation. Why do you think this might be?
3 Assess the fibre content of some food products that are specifically made for children, such as lunchbox products, breakfast cereals.

ACTIVITY

Match the key words below to their correct definitions.

Fibre	Being unable to get rid of solid waste matter easily from the body
Non starch polysaccharide	The name given to a group of plant materials that cannot be digested by humans
Cellulose	The proper scientific name for fibre
Constipation	A plant material that is found in stems, leaves, leaf stalks, the outside layers of seeds and beans, and the peel on fruits and vegetables

PRACTICAL ACTIVITY

Adapt a traditional savoury or sweet dish that would appeal to children to increase the fibre content.

Carry out a nutritional analysis of the recipe to show how the fibre content has been increased.

ASSESSMENT FOR LEARNING

Read the case study below and answer the question at the end.

According to some paediatricians (doctors who specialise in the health of children), many children do not have enough fibre in their diet and suffer from constipation. There are particular concerns about the lack of fruit and vegetables in their diets.

Describe some interesting ways in which fibre could be introduced into the diet of a child who is reluctant to eat fresh fruit and vegetables.

ASSESSMENT FOR LEARNING

Look at the statements below and put a tick ✓ against all the ones you can do. If you can tick them all, well done! Make sure you can remember them in case you are asked to repeat them.

I can...

☐ Describe what fibre is

☐ Explain why the body needs fibre

☐ Name three foods that are good sources of fibre

☐ Identify which types of breakfast cereal have the most fibre

☐ Explain what happens if the body does not have enough fibre

☐ Identify ways of including fibre in the diet.

TOPIC 2

THE RELATIONSHIP BETWEEN DIET AND HEALTH

THE CURRENT DIETARY GUIDELINES

The Eatwell Plate

To help people choose a healthy, balanced diet, health experts and the government have put together a set of eight dietary guidelines:

- Base your meals on starchy foods.
- Eat lots of fruit and vegetables.
- Eat more fish.
- Cut down on saturated fat and sugar.
- Try to eat less salt – no more than 6g a day.
- Get active and try to be a healthy weight.
- Drink plenty of water.
- Do not skip breakfast.

To make the guidelines easier to follow, the Eatwell Plate poster has been produced.

The eatwell plate

Use the eatwell plate to help you get the balance right. It shows how much of what you eat should come from each food group.

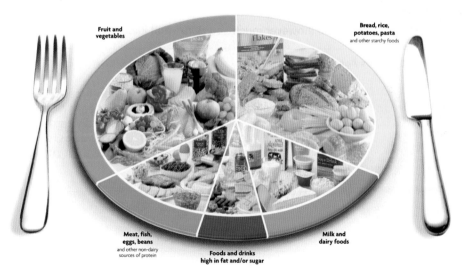

Source: Food Standards Agency

ASSESSMENT FOR LEARNING

1 Why are the green and yellow sections of the Eatwell Plate the biggest?
2 Why is the purple section of the Eatwell plate the smallest?

The guidelines are for most people aged over five years who are in general good health (very young children and babies have their own particular needs). Pregnant women and people with special health conditions have different requirements for food, so the guidelines may not all apply to them.

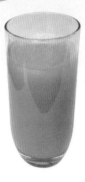

One portion

What do the guidelines mean?

1 **Base your meals on starchy foods**: This means that most of the food on your meal plate should be a starchy plant food, e.g. rice, pasta, potato (but not always chips), bread (preferably wholemeal), oats, millet, cassava, yam and quinoa. These foods will provide you with most of your energy and will also give you a variety of vitamins, minerals and fibre.

2 **Eat lots of fruit and vegetables**: This is to make sure you get a variety of vitamins, minerals, trace elements and fibre, as well as antioxidants and other good natural plant chemicals that we need for good health. Fresh fruit and vegetables are excellent, and frozen and canned varieties also provide nutrients. It is recommended that we eat at least five portions of fruit and vegetables every day, and the Food Standards Agency have produced the following chart to help people work out how much to have.

ONE portion = 80g = any of these

1 apple, banana, pear, orange or other similar sized fruit

2 plums or similar sized fruit

½ a grapefruit or avocado

1 slice of large fruit, such as melon or pineapple

3 heaped tablespoons of vegetables (raw, cooked, frozen or canned)

3 heaped tablespoons of beans and pulses (however much you eat, beans and pulses count as a maximum of one portion a day)

3 heaped tablespoons of fruit salad (fresh or canned in fruit juice) or stewed fruit

1 heaped tablespoon of dried fruit (such as raisins and apricots)

1 handful of grapes, cherries or berries

a dessert bowl of salad

a glass (150ml) of fruit juice (however much you drink, fruit juice counts as a maximum of one portion a day)

Source: Food Standards Agency

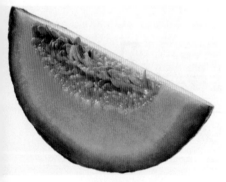

One portion

3 **Eat more fish:** There are three main types of fish as shown in the table below. The guidelines recommend that we eat two portions of fish a week to provide us with a good range of minerals and vitamins as well as protein.

Oily fish also contain omega 3 fatty acids, which are important for the health of the heart. Some canned fish have a lot of salt added, so it is best to eat fresh fish if possible.

Oily fish (oily flesh)	White fish (white, non-oily flesh)	Shellfish (either have a shell or a hard outer skeleton)
Anchovies	Cod	Prawns
Salmon	Haddock	Shrimps
Trout	Plaice	Mussels
Mackerel	Coley	Clams
Herring	Whiting	Squid
Eel	Lemon sole	Crab
Sardines	Skate	Cockles
Pilchards	Halibut	Scallops
Kipper	Rock salmon/dogfish	
Jack fish	Flying fish	
Whitebait	Hake	
Tuna (fresh only)	Hoki	
Swordfish	Pollack	

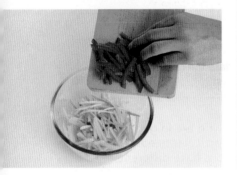

One portion

4a **Cut down on saturated fat:** The guidelines recommend that we eat less food that contains a lot of saturated fats – butter, cheese, cream, coconut oil, palm oil, pastries, cakes, biscuits, chocolate, meat and meat products. A lot of foods have fat 'hidden' in them – the fat is part of the ingredients but you cannot see it. We should eat less high fat foods:

- High fat foods have more than 20g of fat in every 100g of the food.
- Low fat foods have 3g of fat or less in every 100g of the food.

We should eat less saturated fat:

- High saturated fat foods have more than 5g saturates per 100g of the food.
- Low saturated fat foods have 1.5g saturates or less per 100g of the food.

ASSESSMENT FOR LEARNING

The chart below shows how much fat and saturated fat is in some foods.

Name of food	Grams of fat in every 100g of the food	Grams of saturated fat in every 100g of the food
Baked beans in tomato sauce	0.5g	0.08g
Minced beef – average	20.0g	9.0g
Lean minced steak	5.0g	2.5g
Shortbread biscuits	26.0g	15.0g
Wholemeal bread	2.7g	0.5g
Sponge cake	27.0g	10.0g
Cheddar cheese	34.0g	20.0g
Cottage cheese	0.5g	0.25g
Cornish pastie	20.0g	7.0g
Mayonnaise	79.0g	10.0g
Semi skimmed milk	1.5g	0.9g
Sausage roll with flaky pastry	36.0g	14.0g
Sweet potato – boiled	0.6g	0.2g
Shredded wheat	3.0g	0.4g
Sweetcorn	2.0g	0.4g
Yogurt – fruit	1.0g	0.6g
Tuna – canned in oil	22.0g	4.0g
Milk chocolate	30.0g	18.0g
Double cream	48.0g	29.0g
Potato crisps	34.2g (about 8.5g in a 25g bag)	7.0g (about 1.7g in a 25g bag)

1 Identify five foods in the list above that have the highest fat content.
2 Identify five foods in the list above that have the lowest fat content.
3 Identify five foods in the list above that have the highest saturated fat content.
4 Identify five foods in the list above that have the lowest saturated fat content.

Mayonnaise is often used in sandwich fillings to give them flavour, texture and to bind the filling ingredients together so that they do not fall out of the sandwich. Explain why mayonnaise has such a high fat content and suggest some lower fat alternatives that could be used in sandwich fillings instead of mayonnaise.

ASSESSMENT FOR LEARNING

Sam is 25 years old and is trying to change to healthy eating habits, particularly by reducing his fat intake. Look at the list of foods that he usually puts into a lunchbox. Suggest some lower fat alternative foods that Sam could enjoy instead.

- 1 sausage roll
- 1 (25g) packet of crisps
- 2 cheddar cheese and mayonnaise sandwiches
- 2 shortbread biscuits
- 1 apple
- 1 can cola drink

4b **Cut down on sugar:** Most people eat too much sugar. The guidelines recommend that we should have 50 per cent of our daily energy intake from carbohydrate but that only 11 per cent of that amount should come from sugar. Sugar is often 'hidden' in foods and drinks and we do not realise just how much they contain. Even if you look at the ingredients list on a food label, it can be difficult to know how much sugar the food contains because some manufacturers use different chemical names for it, such as glucose, glucose syrup, dextrose, maltose, lactose, fructose, sucrose, invert sugar, hydrolysed starch – these are all sugars!

5 **Try to eat less salt:** Salt has been used for centuries to preserve and flavour foods and we have grown used to its flavour. It is used to make cheese, bacon, ham, bread, yeast extract (e.g. Marmite), peanut butter and smoked fish such as kippers. Many processed foods, especially snack foods, contain a lot of salt, such as cornflakes, potato crisps, roasted salted nuts, savoury fried corn snacks, cracker biscuits, sweet biscuits, pizzas, sausages and cooked meat products. If we eat too much salt it has bad effects on the body:

- It makes your blood pressure rise, which makes your heart have to work harder.
- It puts a strain on your kidneys

ACTIVITY

Look at the drinks below and guess how many teaspoons of sugar each of these contains.

A
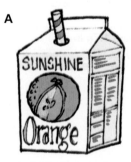
A small carton of orange fruit juice

B
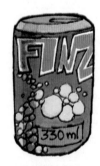
A 330ml can of cola or similar fizzy drink

C
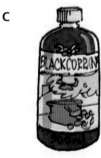
A 500ml bottle of blackcurrant juice drink

D
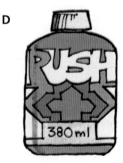
A 380ml bottle of energy juice drink

ACTIVITY

When you are making your own food recipes often tell you to add salt for flavouring. Look at this list of recipes that all suggest you add salt. Suggest some flavourings that you could use instead of salt to help someone who has been told to reduce the amount of salt in their diet.

- Spaghetti Bolognese meat sauce
- Chicken in a white sauce
- Vegetable soup
- Bread rolls
- Tomato sauce for pasta
- Vegetable risotto
- Homemade beef burgers
- Grilled or roasted chicken
- Pan fried white fish

The chemical name for salt is sodium chloride written like this: NaCl. It is the sodium in salt which causes problems in the body. Dietary guidelines recommend that adults have no more than 6g of salt a day (a small teaspoon full). A lot of the salt we eat is 'hidden' as sodium in foods in ingredients such as monosodium glutamate (MSG). This is used as a flavour improver in a lot of ready meals, takeaway foods, savoury snacks and sauces. It is also in sodium bicarbonate which is used as a raising agent in cakes, biscuits, pastries and puddings. It is also found in baking powder and self-raising flour.

6   **Drink plenty of water:** Many people do not drink enough water. Water is essential for the body and we get it from the water we drink and the food we eat.

7   **Do not skip breakfast:** The word 'breakfast' means to break from fasting. Fasting is a period of time when you do not eat. During the night when you sleep, you are fasting and your body is resting. When you wake up, your body is ready to receive food so that it can prepare you for the day's activities ahead. Therefore, breakfast is a very important meal and we should make sure that we give our bodies a good variety of nutrients and energy to set us up for the day. Research has shown that if you eat breakfast, you feel more alert, you can concentrate well and for longer at work or school and you are less likely to eat high fat and sugar snacks later in the morning. Many people do not eat breakfast for a variety of reasons:
- They say they do not have time when getting ready for school or work.
- They say they do not feel hungry.
- They cannot be bothered to prepare food in the morning

There are many breakfast cereal products available to buy, but a lot of them contain large amounts of sugar and salt to give them flavour and make them attractive to children. Many have vitamins and minerals added to them. This is because the natural vitamins and minerals that were found in the cereal grains are destroyed when they are made.

ACTIVITY

Tasty and interesting breakfast food does not have to be complicated or take too long to make. Using foods from the groups listed below, suggest four breakfast menus that would appeal to school children and give them a good start to the day, but would not take long to prepare.

Cereal based: breads, muffins, buns, flour, oats, rice, maize (corn), rye
Dairy foods: eggs, milk, yogurt, butter, cheese
Meat and fish: ham, bacon, white or oily fish
Fruit: fresh fruits, dried fruits, frozen fruits, fruit juices
Vegetables: mushrooms, tomatoes, potatoes, herbs, onions, lentils, beans, etc.

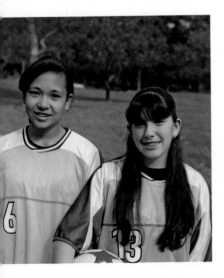

8 **Get active and try to be a healthy weight:** Physical activity is equally important for many reasons:

- It makes you feel good and feel more confident.
- It helps you to maintain a healthy body weight because you balance the energy you take in from food with the energy you use for physical activity.
- It strengthens your bones and helps you grow.
- It makes your heart stronger.
- It makes your digestive system work well.
- It develops your muscles and tones your body which makes you look good.
- It keeps you alert, able to react quickly to situations and to concentrate and learn.
- It boosts your immune system to help you fight disease.
- It reduces your risk of developing some diseases, such as heart disease and cancer.

To be physically active does not mean that you have to be good at sports or spend hours working out in the gym. Everyone can be physically active in their everyday lives by doing things such as:

- walking instead of riding everywhere in a car or on a bus
- walking up stairs rather than using the lift or escalator
- dancing
- housework
- gardening.

To stay healthy and fit, it is recommended that you do some moderate physical activity for 30 minutes at a time, several times a week. It should increase your heart rate so that your breathing becomes heavier (but you can still talk) and make you feel warm.

People who do not do much physical activity are more likely to:

- put on weight
- feel lethargic (tired, weary and not feel like doing anything)
- have weak muscles
- have constipation
- have weak bones
- develop illnesses as they get older.

ASSESSMENT FOR LEARNING

Read the case study below and answer the questions at the end.

Dan is 21 years old and works in an office on the fourth floor of a large business in a busy city centre. He lives one mile away from work and drives his car to the office every day. Dan is becoming concerned because since starting the job a year ago he has put on weight. He does not like how he looks and he feels tired and lethargic most of the time.

1 What changes could Dan make to his lifestyle to help him lose weight, feel livelier and feel better about himself?
2 Plan three appetising main meals that Dan could make for himself that will help him to achieve these goals.

2.1 MAJOR DIET-RELATED HEALTH ISSUES AND CONDITIONS

WHAT IS GOOD HEALTH?

In this topic you will learn about how eating a balanced diet and following a healthy lifestyle helps you to maintain good health. You will also learn about how the body can develop certain health conditions (heart disease, obesity, diabetes, certain cancers) if the diet is not balanced and a healthy lifestyle is not followed.

Being physically healthy is vital for enjoying life. Good physical health results from a mixture of different factors, as shown below.

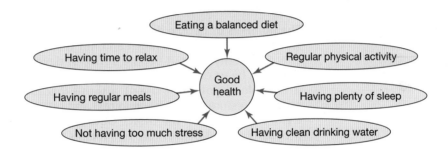

Eating a balanced diet is important because it:

- enables you to grow
- enables you to fight disease
- enables you to be active, alert and to concentrate.

Without a regular supply of a variety of foods, the body would start to deteriorate (become weak) and we would not feel very healthy.

We use the word malnutrition ('mal' means 'bad') to describe what happens when the diet becomes unbalanced and health starts to suffer. Malnutrition can happen when there is not enough food (sometimes called undernutrition) or when there is too much food or too much of one or more nutrients (sometimes called overnutrition).

In the UK and similar countries that follow a diet that has lots of meat, dairy foods, sugar, fats and salt it is unusual to see people with undernutrition, because most people have enough food to eat. But it is more usual to see people with overnutrition because they have too much to eat and do not do enough physical activity.

If malnutrition continues, a person could develop a diet-related health issue or condition. There are several of them linked to overnutrition including:

- obesity
- coronary heart disease
- cardiovascular disease (blood vessels)
- high blood pressure
- diabetes
- osteoporosis
- some cancers.

Each diet-related health issue and condition has a number of risk factors. A risk factor is doing or having something that is more likely to make you develop a disease or health issue / condition. Some risk factors you cannot avoid, such as getting older. But some you can avoid, such as becoming overweight or not being physically active.

In the rest of this topic you will find a description of some diet-related health issues and conditions. Following the description there is a diagram showing the risk factors.

Obesity

Obesity is a health issue in which a person has too much body fat. This is caused by taking in more energy from food than the body uses, so the body converts the excess energy into a store of fat, which builds up over a period of time.

A lot of foods are energy dense (they provide a lot of energy for a small amount of food – usually as fat and sugar), so it is easy to take in more energy than the body needs and many people do not realise how much energy different foods provide.

The numbers of people developing obesity are increasing rapidly throughout the world due to eating too much and not taking enough exercise to use up the energy. Obesity can put people at risk of developing other health conditions, including heart disease, diabetes, some types of cancer, high blood pressure, stroke (blood clot in the brain), arthritis (because of the weight of the body putting pressure on the bone joints) and breathing problems (because of the weight of the fat on the chest). Obesity also causes people to have emotional problems such as depression, and means they are less likely to be able to work.

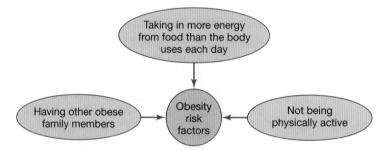

ACTIVITY

1 Identify (list) two risk factors that can lead to obesity.
2 Identify (list) three health conditions that obesity can lead to.

ACTIVITY

There is a lot of concern about childhood obesity and what children eat throughout the day. For example, many foods produced for children's packed lunches are energy dense (cream cheese dips, chocolate bars, fried snacks). Suggest some interesting alternative ideas for foods that could be given to children in their lunch boxes that are less energy dense and provide them with a good variety of nutrients.

Coronary heart disease (CHD)

The heart is a pump, made of muscle, which continually sends blood to all parts of the body. The blood carries oxygen, nutrients and energy to all the body's cells and takes away waste products from them.

To make it work properly, the heart needs its own steady supply of oxygen-rich blood, which flows through the heart's blood vessels (the coronary arteries) to the heart muscle.

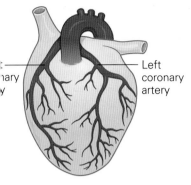

The coronary blood vessels

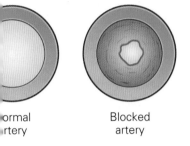

Normal blood vessels and blocked blood vessels

If these coronary arteries get blocked, the heart muscle does not receive enough oxygen, the muscle cannot work and becomes damaged. This causes pain (called angina), and it can lead to a heart attack where part of the heart muscle is permanently damaged. If the heart attack is severe, it can lead to heart failure and death.

In some people the blood vessels in the heart get blocked with fatty substances, which build up if their diet contains a lot of fat, especially saturated fat, which can lead to high blood cholesterol levels. If people smoke cigarettes, substances in the smoke can cause the blood to become 'sticky', which can cause blood clots and blockages in the blood vessels. If a person is overweight, the heart has to work very hard to pump the blood around their body, which can cause a heart attack. If a person eats a lot of salt in their diet, this can cause the blood pressure to rise. This means that the heart has to work harder, which can cause a heart attack.

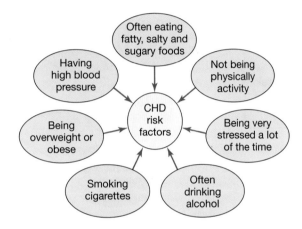

ACTIVITY

1 What do the letters CHD stand for?
2 What substances can block the blood vessels in the heart?
3 What happens to the heart if the blood vessels become blocked?
4 Identify (list) four risk factors that can lead to CHD.

ACTIVITY

1 Suggest a day's menus (breakfast, midday and main meal) for a middle-aged man who is recovering from a heart attack and has been advised by his doctor to change his diet to reduce his fat, sugar and salt intake.
2 Suggest some suitable cooking methods for the following foods to reduce their fat content.
   * Beef burger
   * Potato chips
   * Lamb chop
   * Pork sausages

Cardiovascular disease (CVD)

This health issue includes diseases of the heart and the blood vessels (these are called arteries, capillaries and veins) throughout the body – in the brain, the legs and the lungs. The blood vessels can become blocked anywhere in the body and if this happens, it restricts the amount of oxygen that reaches all the vital organs and tissues. For example, if the blood vessels to the brain become blocked and part of the brain does not receive enough oxygen, the person will have a stroke.

When a stroke happens, the brain cells that have not had enough blood and oxygen are damaged or destroyed. The brain controls everything that happens in the body so having a stroke means that a person will not be able to do certain things, such as talk, do simple tasks like feeding themselves, make simple decisions, move their arms or legs or control their bladder. Elsewhere in the body a restricted blood supply may cause damage to the leg muscles (so it becomes hard to walk), the lungs (so it becomes hard to breathe), the eyes (so it becomes increasingly difficult to see) or the fingers (so it becomes hard to feel and pick up things).

ACTIVITY

1 What happens if blood vessels leading to the brain become blocked?
2 Identify (list) five risk factors that can lead to a stroke.

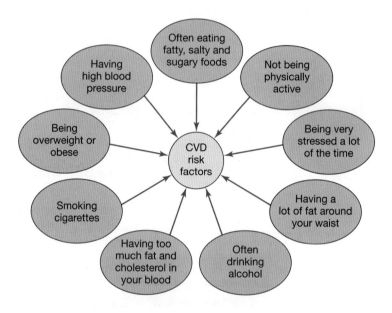

High blood pressure (hypertension)

Blood pressure is the pressure of blood as it passes through your blood vessels. When your blood pressure is taken, the doctor or nurse will take two readings:

The pressure in the arteries when the heart contracts (when it pushes the blood out to send it round the body) – this is called the systolic pressure.

The pressure in the arteries when the heart rests between each heart beat – this is called the diastolic pressure and is a lower number than the first one.

A good blood pressure reading for a healthy, young adult is 110/70 (usually expressed as '110 over 70'). High blood pressure is 140/90 or above.

Blood pressure goes up and down throughout the day. For example, it may be high for a short time if you are stressed, worried or have been exercising, but this does not mean that you have a high blood pressure health condition. People who do have a high blood pressure health condition will have had several high blood pressure readings taken on different occasions and when they are relaxed. There are usually no symptoms if you have high blood pressure, so the only way to check is to have it measured.

Having a high blood pressure health condition means that you are at greater risk of developing CHD and CVD (particularly stroke, eye damage and kidney damage). Blood pressure tends to increase as you get older. Salt intake from food increases blood pressure and there is a lot of concern about the amount of salt that people, especially children, eat everyday (see page 70).

ACTIVITY

1 What is blood pressure?
2 Suggest two situations that can cause blood pressure to go up.
3 What happens to blood pressure as you grow older?
4 Identify (list) four risk factors that can lead to high blood pressure.

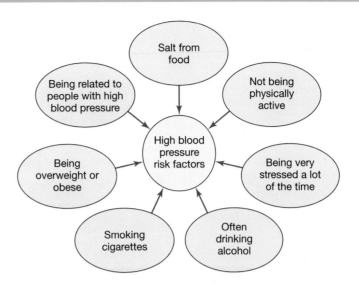

Diabetes

All the cells in our bodies need a constant supply of glucose to enable them to get energy. The glucose is carried to the cells in the blood. To go from the blood and into the cells, the glucose needs a substance called insulin (in the same way that you need a key to unlock a door so that you can go in to a room). Insulin is produced by the pancreas, which is a small body organ, located just behind the stomach.

In some people, this process goes wrong because they have diabetes. This means that they either do not produce any insulin or not enough insulin. The cells cannot get their energy from glucose (because it is 'locked out' and cannot get into the cells) and the glucose stays in the blood, which over a period of time causes damage to the blood vessels. There is no cure for diabetes, but the condition can be controlled.

There are two types of diabetes:

- **Type 1:** This usually develops in children and is due to the pancreas not producing insulin. These diabetics have to have insulin injections every day and eat a carefully balanced diet to control their condition.
- **Type 2**: This is more common than type 1, and used to develop only in older people, but over the past few years many much younger people are developing it because of bad diets and eating habits and being overweight or obese. It happens because although the pancreas produces insulin, the body cells cannot use it, so the glucose cannot get in.

Someone with untreated diabetes will:

- feel thirsty (because of the high levels of glucose in the blood)
- go to the toilet more often because they are drinking more water and because the glucose goes into the urine
- feel tired (because they are not getting any energy from glucose)
- lose weight (because the body will break down fat stores to get energy)
- sometimes get blurred vision.

Eventually diabetes will cause permanent damage in many areas:

- to the eyes (which can lead to blindness)
- the blood vessels in the hands and feet (leading to numbness and the risk of getting infections) and elsewhere in the body
- the skin.

Diabetics do not have to have a very restricted diet. To help control their condition, they should follow the advice on eating from the dietary guidelines and the Eatwell Plate and try to eat regularly throughout the day.

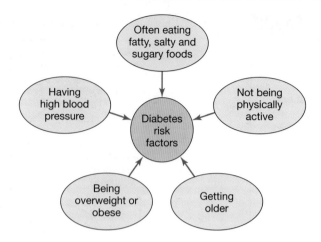

1 Why do the cells in our bodies need glucose?
2 What is the name of the substance that helps glucose go from the blood into the body's cells?
3 Where is insulin produced?
4 What is the health condition that is caused by too much or too little insulin?
5 Describe the two types of diabetes.
6 Identify (list) four risk factors that can lead to a person developing diabetes.

Look at the recipes below and suggest some ways of adapting them to make them more suitable for a person with diabetes.

Name of recipe	Where sugar is used
Sponge cake	In the baked sponge
	In the filling (jam)
	In the topping (icing made with icing sugar and water)
Chocolate chip cookies	In the biscuit mixture
	In the chocolate chips
Fruit crumble and custard	In the stewed fruit
	In the crumble topping
	In the custard

People used to think that diabetics should not have any added sugar in their diet, but now it is thought that they can eat a limited amount of added sugar.

There are various ways in which the amount of added sugar in the diet can be reduced, as the list below shows:

• Reduce the quantity of added sugar in recipes – most recipes will work if the sugar content is reduced.

- Use alternative naturally sweet foods in recipes such as carrots (carrot cake), ripe fresh fruits (bananas, apples, pears, grapes, pineapple), dried fruits (currants, sultanas, apricots, apples, papaya, mango, raisins).
- Use food sweeteners which add flavour but no sugar.

PRACTICAL ACTIVITY

1 Prepare four batches of a traditional all-in-one cake mixture as follows:
   - Batch 1 – use the full amount of sugar stated in the recipe
   - Batch 2 – use 75 per cent of the sugar stated in the recipe
   - Batch 3 – use 50 per cent of the sugar stated in the recipe
   - Batch 4 – use 25 per cent of the sugar stated in the recipe

   Bake the cake mixture as individual cup cakes, but do not add any icing or other topping to them.

   Carry out a tasting panel, where the tasters do not know which batch they are tasting. Ask them to rate the samples for texture, flavour and acceptability.

   Analyse your results to identify which cakes were rated the best and whether reducing the sugar made a noticeable difference to their flavour, texture and acceptability.

2 Adapt a traditional sweet dish to reduce the sugar content.

   Carry out a nutritional analysis to show how the sugar content has been reduced.

Osteoporosis

When we are young, we gradually add minerals (particularly calcium) to our bones to harden and strengthen them. A diet containing a good supply of minerals and doing lots of physical activity (jumping, walking, running, climbing) to stimulate the bones to take up minerals enables this process to take place.

When the bones are full up with minerals, they are said to have reached their peak bone mass ('mass' means how dense the bones are). Most people reach peak bone mass at about 30 to 35 years old. The bones constantly have minerals added and taken away from them to keep the levels of minerals in the blood the same. After peak bone mass is reached, gradually more minerals are taken out of the bones than are put back in to them. This is a natural process of ageing, and it happens in both men and women, but women are more likely to develop it when they reach menopause (this is because they lose the hormones that protect the bones from losing minerals).

The graph shows what happens to the bone mass at different ages.

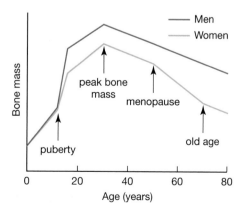

Changes in bone mass with age

Source: Adapted with permission from Medical Research Council Human Nutrition Research

If too much of the minerals are taken out of the bones, the bones become weak, brittle and break easily. This is called osteoporosis (it means bones that are 'porous' – have lots of holes in them) and is a very painful health condition which causes the spine to curve forward making it difficult to walk.

Osteoporosis is usually considered to be a health condition of the elderly, but now there is a lot of concern about younger people developing osteoporosis because they:

- do not do enough physical activity
- do not have enough calcium in their diets
- drink a lot of carbonated (fizzy) drinks such as cola – there is some evidence that suggests that these drinks prevent minerals from being laid down in the bones.

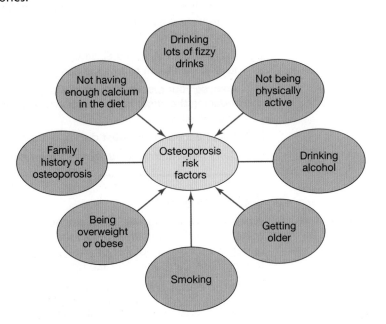

ACTIVITY

Cow's milk contains calcium, and there are also calcium enriched alternative milks such as soya, oat and rice milks. But many children and teenagers prefer to drink sweet fizzy drinks instead of these. Suggest some interesting ways in which milk (any type) can be used in recipes to encourage children and teenagers to increase their calcium intake.

ACTIVITY

1 What is peak bone mass?
2 Look at the graph on the previous page.
   a) At what age is peak bone mass reached for both males and females?
   b) What happens to bone mass for women when they go through the menopause?
   c) Why does this happen? (read the text for the answer)
   d) What happens to bone mass in old age?
   e) Why do you think older people are more likely to suffer bone fractures than younger people?
3 Identify (list) four risk factors that can lead to osteoporosis.

ASSESSMENT FOR LEARNING

Your local health centre is putting up a display about osteoporosis. Design a leaflet that tells people what the risk factors are that can lead to osteoporosis.

On the back of your leaflet, suggest some dishes that contain a good source of calcium or include a recipe suggestion for a dish that is a good source of calcium. Calculate the calcium content of your recipe and include this in your leaflet.

Cancer

Our bodies are made of trillions of cells. Every day new cells are produced to replace cells that have become worn out or damaged. Usually, the body regulates the growth of new cells, but occasionally abnormal cells are produced. Cancer is a growth disorder of abnormal body cells. It starts when a body cell begins to grow in an uncontrolled and invasive way. The result is a cluster of cells, called a tumour, which keeps growing. These abnormal cells do not work properly and if they are not destroyed by the body, they may develop and increase rapidly. The abnormal cells may also spread to other parts of the body and multiply there. Cancer can occur in different parts of the body.

In the UK, the most common cancers in men are lung cancer, prostate cancer and colon cancer. The most common cancers in women are breast cancer, lung cancer and colon cancer (there are many more types).

Cancer is a complicated disease to study for the following reasons:

- It can take many years to develop.
- There are many different forms of cancer.
- A large number of factors are involved.
- Some factors increase the risk of cancer such as smoking cigarettes.
- Some factors reduce the risk of cancer such as eating plenty of fresh fruit and vegetables.
- Some substances can start the process of cancer – these are called carcinogens, such as certain substances in tobacco smoke.
- Some substances affect how fast the cancer develops.

Cancer is a common cause of death in the UK. It is more common in older people than in younger people.

The following things can help to reduce the risk of developing certain types of cancers:

- Eating a healthy, balanced diet with plenty of fruit and vegetables and moderate amounts of red and processed meats.
- Avoiding smoking.
- Keeping alcohol consumption to a moderate level.
- Keeping body weight within the healthy range for height.

ACTIVITY

1 What does cancer mean?
2 Why is cancer a complicated disease to study?
3 List three ways of helping reduce the risk of developing cancer.
4 Identify (list) three risk factors for developing cancer.

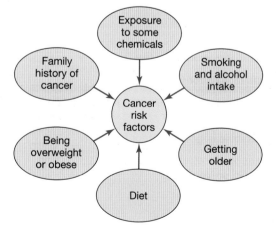

WHY ARE SO MANY PEOPLE DEVELOPING DIET-RELATED HEALTH ISSUES?

There is a lot of concern about the numbers of people who are developing diet-related health issues, especially in countries such as the UK and America. For example, every year in the UK:

- Approximately 208,000 people die from heart disease.

ASSESSMENT FOR LEARNING

When you have worked through Topic 2.1, look at the statements below for each diet-related health issue or condition and put a tick ✓ against all the ones you can do. If you can tick them all, well done! Make sure you can remember them in case you are asked to repeat them.

I can...

☐ Explain what 'malnutrition' and 'over nutrition' mean

☐ Describe how the body benefits from having good physical health

☐ Name three factors for achieving good physical health

☐ Identify three foods that are eaten in large amounts in the diet of people in the UK

☐ Explain what a risk factor is

☐ Identify why it is important to have a balanced diet

Obesity: I can...

☐ Describe what obesity is

☐ Explain how the body is affected by obesity

☐ Name three risk factors for obesity

☐ Identify three types of foods that are energy dense

☐ Explain what other health conditions are linked to obesity

☐ Identify why more people are developing obesity

Coronary heart disease: I can...

☐ Describe what CHD is

☐ Explain how the heart is affected by CHD

☐ Name three risk factors for CHD

☐ Identify why it is important to limit your intake of saturated fat

☐ Explain why exercise is good for your heart

☐ Identify the importance of eating fruit and vegetables to help prevent CHD

Cardiovascular disease: I can...

☐ Describe what CVD is

☐ Explain how the body is affected by CVD

☐ Name three risk factors for CVD

☐ Identify three foods that have a high salt content

High blood pressure: I can...

☐ Describe what blood pressure is and how it is measured

☐ Explain how the body is affected by high blood pressure

☐ Name three risk factors for high blood pressure

☐ Identify which type of foods may increase blood pressure

☐ Explain what happens if a person has a stroke

Diabetes: I can...

☐ Describe what diabetes is and the difference between the two types

☐ Explain how the body is affected by diabetes

☐ Name three risk factors for diabetes

☐ Identify three symptoms of untreated diabetes

☐ Explain what type of diet a diabetic person should follow

Osteoporosis: I can...

☐ Describe what osteoporosis is

☐ Explain how the body is affected by osteoporosis

☐ Name three risk factors for osteoporosis

☐ Identify three symptoms of osteoporosis

☐ Explain what peak bone mass is

☐ Identify why it is important to have enough calcium in the diet and be physically active when you are young

- Approximately 2.6 million people have heart disease but are still alive.
- Approximately 1.8 million people have type 2 diabetes and another 1 million have it but have not yet been diagnosed – these figures are increasing rapidly.

There is particular concern about the large numbers of children and young people who are developing these issues.

There are a number of reasons why so many people are developing diet-related health issues:

- Food and eating habits have changed dramatically over the past 50 years. Many countries now have what is known as a western diet, which contains a lot of red meat, dairy foods, fried foods, refined carbohydrate (white flour, white sugar) and additives. There is also less fruit and vegetables and fewer raw, unprocessed foods.
- Many people eat lots of snacks throughout the day rather than sitting down to regular set meals. Many snack foods contain a lot of fat, sugar and salt.
- Many people eat processed foods and ready-made meals rather than cook for themselves. Such foods often contain a lot of fat, sugar, salt and additives.
- There are many foods to choose from and a lot of people eat more than their body needs each day.
- People eat out at restaurants and fast food places. The foods and drinks sold there are often energy dense and the portion sizes are often large.
- Many people do not regularly eat fresh fruits and vegetables.
- People are generally much less active than they used to be:
  - They do not walk because they drive cars or ride on a bus.
  - They sit at a desk using a computer at work all day.
  - They watch a lot of television or play computer games.
  - They have machines to do work for them.
  - They live in heated homes so they do not need to be active to stay warm.

2.2 ADAPTING MEALS AND DIETS

FOLLOWING THE DIETARY GUIDELINES

If people want to follow the dietary guidelines, it is easy to make a series of small changes to adapt meals and diets and still enjoy food.

Here is a reminder of the dietary guidelines:

- Base your meals on starchy foods.
- Eat lots of fruit and vegetables.
- Eat more fish.
- Cut down on saturated fat and sugar.
- Try to eat less salt – no more than 6g a day.
- Get active and try to be a healthy weight.
- Drink plenty of water.
- Do not skip breakfast.

Buying your food

Here is some good advice on how to buy food:

- Learn to read and understand food labels, especially the nutrition information so that you can make informed choices when you buy food.
- Also use the guidance systems on food labels, such as the 'Traffic Lights' one designed by the Food Standards Agency (shown below).
- Make a list of the foods you need to buy and try to stick to it, so that you do not buy less healthy foods on impulse.
- Try not to shop for food when you are hungry because you might be tempted to buy food you had not planned to eat.

In the Traffic Lights scheme, the colours have the following meanings:
- **Red:** the food is HIGH in fat, salt or sugar.
- **Amber:** the food is not too high or low in fat, salt or sugar.
- **Green:** the food is LOW in fat, salt or sugar.

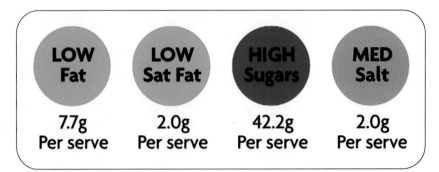

Source: Food Standards Agency

Preparing your food

If you are using a recipe, have a look at the list of ingredients and see if you can reduce any ingredients, such as the fat, sugar or salt. Add any ingredients (extra fruit or vegetables) or change any ingredient (use wholemeal flour for extra fibre or use a reduced fat dairy product).

When you are preparing your food, pay attention to the amount of fat (oil), salt and sugar you add – you may find that you are adding a lot more than you actually need to.

Cooking your food

It may be possible to change the cooking method you are using to reduce the amount of fat in the food. For example, grilling meat instead of frying it will let the fat in the meat drain away, poaching or boiling an egg instead of frying will avoid using fat and oven baking chips instead of frying them will reduce their fat content.

When stir-frying vegetables, meat or poultry, if the pan starts to become dry, add a little water instead of more oil. The water will bubble and steam and moisten the food so that it does not burn and you will not have added extra fat to the pan.

If you are cooking food for someone who does not like vegetables very much, 'disguise' them by cooking them and then pureeing them to add to sauces or soups or meat dishes such as stews.

If you are frying a food in oil, make sure that the oil is hot enough to start cooking the food as soon as it is put in the pan. If the oil is too cool, the food will sit in it and soak up the oil before it starts to cook, which will increase the amount of fat it contains. When the food is cooked place it on some kitchen towel to soak up any excess oil.

Use alternative flavours to salt for savoury recipes – herbs (fresh or dried), spices (fresh or dried), vegetables such as onion, celery and garlic, and fruits such as lemon, orange or lime zest and juice.

ACTIVITY

Your local supermarket has asked you to design a leaflet for them to display at the checkout. The leaflet is to be about how people can adapt meals and diets.

Use the information above to help you design your leaflet. Include some information on buying, preparing and cooking food. Remember to pick out a few key points for each part. Make your leaflet attractive so customers will pick it up and read it.

Here are some ways in which you can reduce the fat, sugar or salt in food.

Your aim	Suggestions for how to do it
REDUCE fat	• Choose lean cuts of meat. • When buying minced meat, check on the label for the fat content and try to buy minced meat that has no more than 5 per cent fat. • Trim the fat from meat and poultry before cooking. • Grill or oven bake foods such as meat, sausages and fish rather than fry them in fat or oil (because the fat will melt and drain away from the food). • When shallow frying or stir frying food, if the food starts to become dry, add a little water rather than more oil to continue the cooking. • Choose low or reduced fat versions of foods such as yogurt, cheese, milk, biscuits and low fat spreads. • Reduce the amount of butter or margarine that you spread on bread. • Instead of using mayonnaise in sandwiches or to mix salad ingredients, try using low fat versions of crème fraiche, salad dressing or fromage frais instead. • Buy canned oily fish such as tuna and sardines in tomato sauce, water or brine instead of oil. • Instead of adding butter or margarine to mashed potato, add wholegrain mustard. • Instead of eating ice cream, try sorbet which has a low fat content.
REDUCE salt	• Use alternative flavours to salt when cooking – spices, herbs, pepper. • Cut down the amounts of foods that have salt added to them such as cheeses, processed meats, salted fish, yeast extract and savoury snack foods (crisps). • Buy reduced salt versions of foods such as canned fish, crisps, canned beans. • Read labels and check for ingredients other than salt that contain sodium, such as monosodium glutamate, bicarbonate of soda and baking powder. • Check labels for foods such as breads, breakfast cereals and bottled water which sometimes have quite a lot of added sodium. • Eat naturally low salt foods such as fruits and vegetables.
REDUCE sugar	• Reduce the quantity of added sugar in recipes – most recipes will work if the sugar content is reduced. • Use alternative naturally sweet foods in recipes such as carrots (carrot cake), ripe fresh fruits (bananas, apples, pears, grapes, pineapple), dried fruits (currants, sultanas, apricots, apples, papaya, mango, raisins). • Use food sweeteners which add flavour but no sugar.
INCREASE fibre and fruit and vegetable intake	• Eat whole grain (wholemeal) breakfast cereals, bread, rice and pasta. • Use wholemeal flour (either all wholemeal or half wholemeal and half white) for recipes such as cakes, scones, pastries, biscuits, bread, crumbles, sponge puddings. • Add oat or wheat bran to crumble toppings, cake, pastry and biscuit recipes. • Add chopped fresh or dried fruits to your breakfast cereal. • Add chopped dried fruits to cake, scone and biscuit recipes. • Eat porridge for breakfast and add stewed fruit such as apples, plums and prunes. • Eat plenty of fresh fruits, salads and vegetables, and leave the skins on where you can. • Make delicious fruit smoothies with a blender, using a variety of fresh fruits. • Eat dried fruits as snacks. • Add peas, beans and lentils to stews, soups, curries. • Add finely chopped vegetables to dishes such as Bolognese and curry. • Make soups using a variety of vegetables – these can be blended or chunky. • Add seeds to crumbles, breads, stews, soups, breakfast cereals, biscuit and cake mixtures.

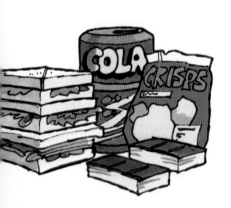

Menu 2

ASSESSMENT FOR LEARNING

Set out below are some menus for meals for different people.

For each meal explain what you would change with a reason why.

Then make suggestions on how you would adapt the menu or any of the recipes in it to make the meal follow more closely the dietary guidelines.

Menus 1, 2 and 3: For an average adult who is not very physically active

1 Breakfast

- Large bowl of sugar coated cornflakes and whole milk
- A large croissant spread with butter and jam
- A cup of tea with four teaspoons of sugar added

2 Midday meal

- Four sandwiches made with white bread and filled with butter, ham, mayonnaise and cheese
- A packet of potato crisps
- Two chocolate wafer biscuits
- A can of cola drink

3 Evening meal

- Fried chicken curry (includes onion and canned tomatoes) served with white rice
- Large slice of apple pie with ice cream and custard

Menus 4, 5 and 6: For an eight-year-old child

4 Breakfast

- Small bowl of chocolate coated cereal with milk
- Glass of orange squash

5 Midday meal

- A small pot of cheese spread and four very small bread sticks
- A chocolate bar
- A small carton of blackcurrant drink

6 Evening meal

- Four fried chicken nuggets
- A portion of potato chips
- A portion of baked beans
- A small fruit flavoured yogurt

Menus 7, 8 and 9: For a teenage girl

7 Breakfast

- None
- A can of cola on the way to school

8 Midday meal

- A portion of chips
- A doughnut
- A can of fizzy orange drink

9 Evening meal

- Two fried sausages
- Mashed potato
- Peas
- Portion of ice cream and chocolate sauce

Menus 10, 11 and 12: For a middle-aged woman who needs to lose weight

10 Breakfast
- A fried bacon roll
- A glass of orange juice
- Two slices of toast with marmalade

11 Midday meal
- An omelet made with four eggs and cheese
- A small bowl of salad with mayonnaise
- A slice of fruit cake with marzipan and icing on it

12 Evening meal
- A medium-sized beef steak, fried with onions and mushrooms
- A baked potato with butter and cream cheese
- A grilled tomato
- A slice of cheesecake with ice cream

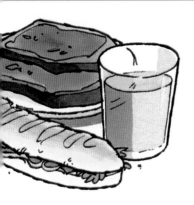

Menu 10

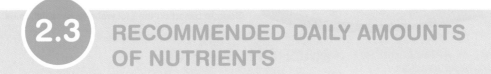

2.3 RECOMMENDED DAILY AMOUNTS OF NUTRIENTS

DIETARY REFERENCE VALUES

You have now learned about nutrients and why they are so important for growth and good health. You have also learned that there are guidelines about how much of different foods we should eat every day in order to grow properly and stay healthy, and what happens if we do not eat a balanced diet.

The guidelines are based on information that has been put together by scientists and health professionals, who have worked out how much of each nutrient our bodies need. They have called this information dietary reference values (DRVs).

DRVs show the amount of energy and nutrients that different groups of people need for growth and good health. The groups are based on age, gender (male or female) and for females during pregnancy and lactation (breastfeeding).

DRVs only apply to healthy people. They do not apply to people who have a disease or a health issue or condition, because the body's needs for nutrients and energy change under these conditions.

DRVs are used for guidance only. They are based on the needs of an average person and so they do not apply to everyone, but they are very helpful to people who have to provide food for groups of people – in schools, hospitals, residential homes and prisons – to make sure they provide nutritionally balanced meals.

The figures that are given for each nutrient are meant to be enough for the needs of about 97 per cent of a group of people.

Food manufacturers and retailers often show DRVs as guideline daily amounts (GDAs), which may appear on the label at the front of a food product, as shown on the left.

There is often a more detailed explanation of what this means on the nutritional information elsewhere on the label, as in the one overleaf.

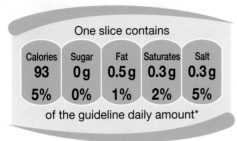

One slice contains

Calories	Sugar	Fat	Saturates	Salt
93	0g	0.5g	0.3g	0.3g
5%	0%	1%	2%	5%

of the guideline daily amount*

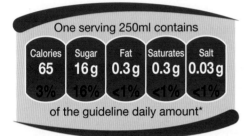

One serving 250ml contains

Calories	Sugar	Fat	Saturates	Salt
65	16g	0.3g	0.3g	0.03g
3%	16%	<1%	<1%	<1%

of the guideline daily amount*

Typical values per 100g of the foodstuff → Per 100g

Typical values per portion (e.g. slice) of the product → Per slice 50g

GDA: Guideline Daily Amount per portion → % GDA

Typical values	Per 100g	Per slice 50g	% GDA
Energy	776 kJ/185 kcal	388 kJ/93 kcal	5%
Protein	7.0g	3.5g	7%
Carbohydrates	37g	19g	7%
Of which sugars	0g	0g	0%
Fat	1.0g	0.5g	1%
Of which saturates	0.5g	0.3g	2%
Fibre	5.0g	2.5g	10%
Sodium	0.2g	0.1g	4%
Salt equivalent	0.6g	0.3g	5%
GDA = adult's daily guideline amount			

Source: based on the Lidl website www.lidl.co.uk

MACRONUTRIENTS

The table opposite gives the DRVs for protein and energy. The figures for energy are averages, because the amount of energy required depends very much on how physically active people are.

ACTIVITY

1 How much protein does a 17-year-old boy need?
2 How much protein does a 17-year-old girl need?
3 Can you explain why a boy needs more protein?
4 Can you explain why pregnant and lactating women need extra protein?

ACTIVITY

1 How many Kcals does a 16-year-old boy need?
2 How many Kcals does a 16-year-old girl need?
3 Can you explain why there is a difference between these figures for boys and girls?

Fat and carbohydrate

DRVs for these two nutrients are given as a percentage (%) of daily energy intake for adults. 1

Nutrient	% of daily energy that should come from this nutrient
Fat	35%
Added sugar	11%
Starch and natural sugars in food	39%
Total carbohydrate	11% + 39% = 50%
Fibre	Minimum 18g per day (30g per day is recommended)

Age		Protein DRV (grams)	Energy (kJ)	Energy (kcal)
Male				
0–3 months		12.5	2,280	545
1–3 years		14.5	5,150	1,230
7–10 years		28.3	8,240	1,970
11–14 years		42.1	9,270	2,220
15–18 years		55.2	11,510	2,755
19–50 years		55.5	10,600	2,550
50+ years	51–59 years	53.3	10,600	2,550
	60–64 years		9,930	2,380
	65–74 years		9,710	2,330
	75+ years		8,770	2,100
Female				
0–3 months		12.5	2,160	515
4–6 months		12.7	2,690	645
7–9 months		13.7	3,200	765
10–12 months		14.9	3,610	865
1–3 years		14.5	4,860	1,165
4–6 years		19.7	6,460	1,545
7–10 years		28.3	7,280	1,740
11–14 years		41.2	7,920	1,845
15–18 years		45.0	8,830	2,110
19–50 years		45.0	8,100	1,940
50+ years	51–59 years	46.5	8,000	1,904
	60–64 years		7,990	1,902
	65–74 years		7,960	1,895
	75+ years		7,610	1,810
During pregnancy		Add another 6g	Add 840 kJ	Add 200 kcal
During lactation		Add another 11g	Add 1,900 kJ	Add 450 kcal

MICRONUTRIENTS

The DRVs for micronutrients are given on the next page in milligrams or micrograms, depending on the nutrients. A milligram (mg) is a thousandth of a gram: 1/1,000g. A microgram (µg) is a millionth of a gram: 1/1,000,000g.

ACTIVITY

1 How much vitamin B_1 does a 13-year-old boy need?
2 How much vitamin B_1 does a 13-year-old girl need?
3 Can you think why a boy needs more vitamin B_1?

Age	Vit. B$_1$ (thiamin) (mg)	Vit. B$_2$ (riboflavin) (mg)	Vit. B$_3$ (niacin) (mg)	Vit. B$_6$ (pyridoxine) (mg)	Vit. B$_9$ (folate) (µg)	Vit. B$_{12}$ (cobalamin) (µg)	Vit. C (ascorbic acid) (mg)	Vit. A (retinol) (µg)	Vit. D (cholecalciferol) (µg)*	Calcium (mg)	Iron (mg)**	Sodium (mg)	Iodine (mg)
0–3 months	0.2	0.4	3	0.2	50	0.3	25	350	8.5	525	1.7	210	50
4–6 months											4.3	280	60
7–10 months	0.3		5	0.3		0.4			7.0		7.8	320	
10–12 months												350	
1–3 years	0.5	0.6	8	0.4	70	0.5	30	400		350	6.9	500	70
4–6 years	0.7	0.8	11	0.9	100	0.8			8.5	450	6.1	700	100
7–10 years		1.0	12	1.0	150	1.0		500	0–10	550	8.7	1200	110
Male													
11–14 years	0.9	1.2	15	1.2	200	1.2	35	600	0–10	1000	11.3	1600	130
15–18 years		1.3	18	1.5		1.5	40	700					140
19–50 years			17	1.4						700	8.7		
50+ years			16						10 (at 65+ years)				
Female													
11–14 years	0.7	1.1	12	1.0	200	1.2	35	600	0–10	800	14.8	1600	130
15–18 years	0.8		14	1.2		1.5	40						140
19–50 years			13							700			
50+ years			12						10 (at 65+ years)		8.7		
During pregnancy	Add 0.1	Add 0.3	No extra	No extra	Add 100	No extra	Add 10	Add 100	10	No extra	No extra	No extra	No extra
During lactation	Add 0.2	Add 0.5	Add 2		Add 60	Add 0.5	Add 30	Add 350		Add 550			

*Above the age of 4, vitamin D requirements vary depending on how much exposure the skin has to sunlight.

** Adult females may need a larger quantity of iron if they lose a lot of blood during periods; during pregnancy if advised by a doctor; or during lactation if a lot of blood was lost during childbirth.

ACTIVITY

1 How much vitamin B_2 does a 13-year-old boy need?
2 How much vitamin B_2 does a 13-year-old girl need?
3 Can you think why a boy needs more vitamin B_2?

ACTIVITY

1 How much vitamin B_3 does a 17-year-old boy need?
2 How much vitamin B_3 does a 17-year-old girl need?
3 Can you think why a boy needs more vitamin B_3?

ACTIVITY

1 How much vitamin B_6 does a 15-year-old boy need?
2 How much vitamin B_6 does a 15-year-old girl need?
3 Can you think why a boy needs more vitamin B_6?

ACTIVITY

1 How much vitamin B_9 does a 19-year-old woman need?
2 How much vitamin B_9 does a 19-year-old pregnant woman need?
3 Can you think why a pregnant woman needs more vitamin B_9?

ACTIVITY

1 How much vitamin B_{12} does a 13-year-old boy need?
2 How much vitamin B_{12} does a 73-year-old man need?
3 Can you think why an elderly man needs more vitamin B_{12} than a boy?

ACTIVITY

1 How much vitamin C does a 19-year-old woman need?
2 How much vitamin C does a 19-year-old pregnant woman need?
3 Can you think why a pregnant woman needs more vitamin C?

ACTIVITY

1 How much vitamin A does a 19-year-old woman need?
2 How much vitamin A does a 19-year-old lactating woman need?
3 Can you think why a lactating woman needs more vitamin A?

ENERGY AND FOOD

WHAT IS ENERGY?

Energy gives us the ability to do work, move around, keep warm and be active. We need a certain amount of energy just to stay alive and keep everything in the body working – the heart beating, the digestive system working and the brain sending out messages to the body. This amount is called the basal metabolic rate (BMR).

How is energy used in the body?

Energy is used all the time for various jobs in the body.

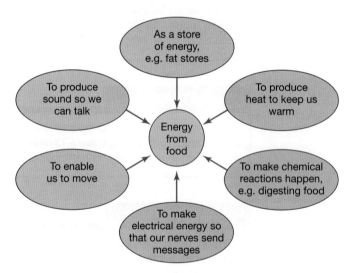

The amount of energy that different people require varies from day to day. The factors that influence how much energy you need are:

- **Your age:** Babies and children need a lot of energy because they are usually very active and are continually growing. Teenagers need more energy than adults because they are still growing and are often (but not always!) very active. As people get older, their energy requirements gradually get smaller as the body starts to slow down.
- **Your activity levels:** The more physically active you are, the more energy you will use. Some activities – athletics, playing rugby or football, manual building work, working in a job where you are continually lifting heavy objects, climbing mountains and cycling long distances – use up large amounts of energy and people have to make sure that they eat enough energy-dense food at regular intervals throughout the day to sustain them.
- **Your state of health:** Sometimes an illness may increase your energy use as your body tries to fight an infection. The illness may stop you being physically active and it may reduce your appetite, so your body will have to rely on getting energy from its fat stores. This is why people often find they lose weight when they have been ill. When a woman is pregnant or lactating (breastfeeding her baby), her energy needs will increase to cope with the demands of the growing baby on her body.

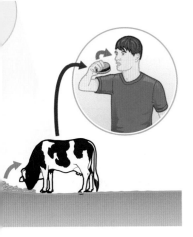

Where energy comes from

• **Your gender:** On average, males need more energy each day than females because they are generally bigger and have more muscles (muscles use a lot of energy). Everyone has individual needs for energy, so a tall, physically active female will use more energy than a short, non-active male!

Where does energy come from?

All energy originally comes from the sun. Plants trap the sun's energy and store it as carbohydrate (sugars and starch) or fat. Animals eat the plants and use some of the energy from them to be active and store some of it as fat. People eat animals and plants and use the energy that is found in the macronutrients they contain (carbohydrates, fats and proteins).

HOW IS ENERGY MEASURED?

Energy is measured in two ways:

• We use a metric unit called the joule (J). One joule is a very small measurement, so for measuring energy in food we use the kilojoule (kJ).
• We also use another measurement called the calorie (cal). One calorie is a very small measurement, so for measuring energy in food we use the kilocalorie (kcal).
  1 kJ = 1,000J
  1 kcal = 1,000cal
  1 kcal = 4.2kJ

SOURCES OF ENERGY

Our bodies prefer to use carbohydrate as the main source of energy. During digestion, the carbohydrate is broken down into individual glucose molecules. Glucose travels round the bloodstream to all the body cells to provide them with energy. Some of the glucose is stored as glycogen in the liver and muscles to provide the body with an easily available supply of energy, e.g. for running.

Fat is also used as a source of energy, but it has to be changed into glucose in the body first. Our bodies store fat under the skin in adipose tissue so we can use it if we do not have enough to eat.

The body prefers to use protein for body growth and repair, but it will use it for energy if there is not enough carbohydrate or fat. To do this, it has to change the protein to glucose.

Different foods have different energy values. It is possible to measure this in a laboratory using special equipment. Lists of the energy values of lots of different foods are available in books, on special computer programs and on the internet.

The energy values for the three main sources of energy in the diet are shown below.

<table>
<tr><td>ACTIVITY</td></tr>
<tr><td>1 How is energy measured?
2 Name two nutrients that are good sources of energy.</td></tr>
</table>

Source of energy	Energy value	
	kJ	kcal
1g of pure **carbohydrate**	15.7	3.75
1g of pure **fat**	37.8	9.0
1g of pure **protein**	16.8	4.0

Alcohol also provides the body with energy. 1g of pure alcohol has an energy value of 29.4 kJ/7 kcal.

Some foods are energy dense. This means that they will provide a lot more energy than the same weight of another food, which is a low energy food. Here are some examples of energy dense and low energy foods.

Name of food	Weight	kJ	kcal
Milk chocolate bar	100g	2177	520
Potato crisps	100g	2215	530
Pork pie	100g	1514	363
Cornish pasty	100g	1117	267
Cheesecake	100g	1769	426
Green salad	100g	51	12
Salad with nuts and mayonnaise	100g	1056	278
Honeydew melon	100g	119	28
Orange	100g	158	37
Grilled cod fish	100g	402	95

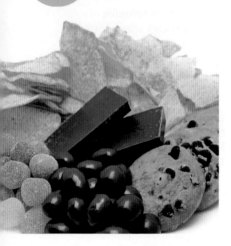

Energy-dense foods

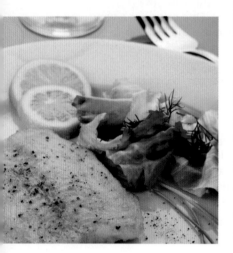

Low-energy foods

ACTIVITY

1 Which three foods in the chart above are the most energy dense? Explain why.
2 Which three foods in the chart above are the least energy dense? Explain why.

WHAT INFLUENCES AN INDIVIDUAL'S ENERGY REQUIREMENTS?

To understand what influences individual energy requirements we need to look at how energy is released from food into the body.

In every living cell in the body, energy is gradually released in a series of small steps. This is called respiration. This happens all the time so that we have a constant supply of energy.

We use oxygen to release the energy from food in our bodies. We get the oxygen from breathing it in through our lungs. When energy has been released, water is produced, some of which is used by the body. We also breathe out carbon dioxide gas and water (you can see this as you breathe on to a cold window or mirror).

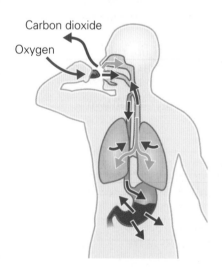

Carbon dioxide

Oxygen

ACTIVITY

1 Identify (list) three uses of energy in the body.
2 Suggest three factors that can influence an individual's energy requirements.
3 Why do babies and children need a lot of energy?
4 Why do teenagers need more energy than adults?
5 Name two activities that use up a lot of energy.
6 Give one reason why a builder might need more energy than an office worker.

Energy intake and expenditure

Most of the energy we need every day comes from the food we eat. We can store energy in the body:

- as glycogen in the liver and muscles (for a quick burst of energy – when you suddenly run)
- as fat in special tissue under the skin called adipose tissue (to supply the body with energy if not enough comes from food).

As noted at the beginning of this topic, we need a certain amount of energy just to stay alive and keep everything in the body working – the heart beating, the digestive system working and the brain sending out messages to the body. This amount is called the basal metabolic rate (BMR).

We also need more energy for any physical activity that we do – walking, standing, nodding our head, talking and picking up a bag.

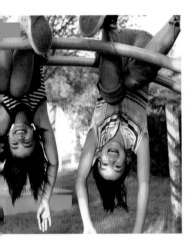

Energy balance

Over a period of time, if we take in the same amount of energy each day that we use for all body activities, our weight will stay constant (the same). If we take in less energy each day than we use for all body activities, we will use energy from our fat stores and we will lose weight. And if we take in more energy each day than we use for all body activities, we will store the extra as fat and we will gain weight.

When we are young, our energy requirements are high as the body is growing and we tend to be very active. Active children usually have a healthy body weight. However, there is concern that a lot of children and teenagers do not have enough physical activity because they spend a lot of time watching television, using computers and being driven around in cars. These children are likely to become overweight if their energy intake is more than their physical activity.

As we get older, our energy requirements gradually decrease as the body slows down.

ACTIVITY

1 How is energy stored in the body?
2 What happens over a period of time if we take in more energy than we use for all our body activities?
3 A friend of yours has taken up running and swimming. She does these every day for at least an hour. She has cut down on what she eats, especially sugary and high fat foods. What is likely to happen to her weight?
4 Why will this happen?

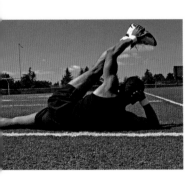

Physical activity

Some physical activities use a lot of energy, such as running, climbing stairs, swimming, digging, lifting heavy weights and cycling. Some physical activities use very little energy, such as sitting in a chair, watching television, driving a car and using a computer.

People who are very physically active need to make sure they eat enough food to give them the energy they need so that they maintain their weight. For example, an athlete who weighs 50kg and trains for four hours a day will need approximately 13,692 kJ/3,260 kcals each day to maintain their body weight.

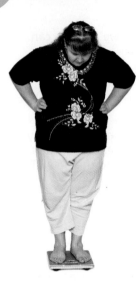

Physically inactive (sedentary) people need to make sure that they do not have more energy from their food each day than they use, to avoid gaining weight. For example, a sedentary person in their mid-20s weighing 50kg will need approximately 7,266 kJ/1,730 kcal each day to maintain their body weight.

People who have gained too much weight and want to lose some of it need to make sure that they take in less energy than they use and increase their physical activity, so that their body uses up its fat stores.

This process will not happen quickly and will require determination and perseverance! It takes time to become overweight so it will take time to lose the weight. For example, an overweight person in their mid-20s who weighs 100kg and wants to lose weight will need to increase their daily physical activity levels and take in approximately 6,384 kJ/1,520 kcal per day in order to lose about 0.5 to 1kg per week (which is what is advised as a sensible rate of weight loss).

ACTIVITY

Match each word with its correct definition by drawing arrows between each of the charts.

Energy dense	The amount of energy that a food can supply to the body
Physical activity	The process by which energy is released from food in small steps using oxygen
Energy	The amount of energy needed by the body just to stay alive
Energy balance	Making the body work so that it uses more energy than just the amount needed to stay alive
Basal metabolic rate	Foods that supply a lot of energy compared to the same weight of a low energy food
Respiration	Taking in the right amount of energy from food to match the body's energy requirements
Energy value	The ability of the body to do work, move, keep warm and be active

ASSESSMENT FOR LEARNING

Read the case study below and answer the questions at the end.

Maggie and Leon are in their early 20s and both work in sedentary office jobs. They have decided that they want to improve their long-term health by increasing their physical activity levels and reducing their daily energy intake. This has increased over the last few months due to both of them eating a lot of takeaway and ready meals, energy dense snack foods and alcoholic and sweetened drinks.

Here is a typical day's food intake for each of them.

Maggie	Leon
Breakfast: One fried bacon sandwich Cup of coffee with cream and sugar **Mid morning snack:** Three chocolate digestive biscuits Cup of coffee with cream and sugar **Lunch:** Hot meat pasty and a cream doughnut Can of cola drink **After work:** Chocolate bar **Evening meal:** Two glasses of wine Fried fish and chips with peas Bowl of ice cream	**Breakfast:** Two fried bacon sandwiches Cup of tea with sugar **Mid morning snack:** Large piece of fruit cake Cup of coffee with cream and sugar **Lunch:** Large burger with fries and a vanilla thick shake **After work:** Large bag of potato crisps **Evening meal:** Three glasses of wine Fried fish and chips with peas Bowl of ice cream and chocolate sauce

1 Using the daily food intake examples above, explain how Maggie and Leon could make their daily food intake less energy dense.
2 Plan three lunch and evening meals for the couple to help them with their change in lifestyle and eating habits. Explain how the menu will help them to balance their energy intake.
3 What might be the consequences for the couple's long-term health if they do not alter their eating habits and current levels of physical activity?

TOPIC

4

FOOD COMMODITIES

  MEAT AND POULTRY

Meat and poultry are an important part of the diet for people in many countries. Meat comes from animals, and poultry is the name for meat from birds.

NUTRITIONAL VALUE

Animal meat and poultry meat have a similar structure (they are in fact muscles) and nutrients, but the amount of each nutrient varies according to the following:

- the age of the animal or bird
- the part of the animal or bird that is eaten
- how the animal or bird is reared (where it is housed, what it is fed on, how much it can move around, how quickly it grows, how much muscle and fat it builds up).

Cooking the meat and poultry helps to make the nutrients more digestible and easier for the body to absorb. (see page 196).

Meat and poultry provide the following nutrients:

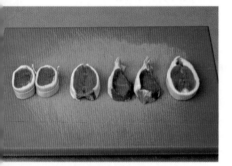

- **Protein:** Meat and poultry provide an important source of high biological value protein. Offal (liver) is a good source of HBV protein which is easily digested.
- **Fat:** Meat and poultry both provide fat, much of which is saturated. The fat is found under the skin and inbetween the muscle fibres. Meat tends to have more fat than poultry, but birds which have been reared in large numbers in sheds (called intensive farming) often have a high fat content because they cannot move around much to use it up for energy. There is less fat in offal than in muscle meat.
- **Fat soluble vitamins A and D:** Meat and poultry provide some of these. The amount varies according to how much fat they contain and what they have eaten. Liver is a very rich source of vitamin A, but pregnant women are advised not to eat it in early pregnancy as the high levels may cause birth defects. Kidney and heart also contain vitamin A.

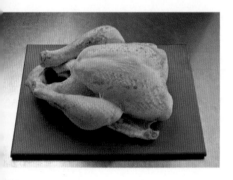

- **Group B vitamins:** Meat and poultry are both good sources of B vitamins. Heart and liver contain useful amounts of vitamin B1.
- **Iron:** Red meat is an important source of iron. Meat and poultry also provide a range of trace elements. Liver is an important source of iron.
- **Water:** Meat and poultry naturally contain water, and sometimes extra water is added to them by food processors.

ACTIVITY

1 What type of protein do meat, poultry and offal contain?
2 Where is the fat found in meat?
3 Why does some intensively reared poultry, such as chicken, have more fat than free range poultry?
4 Why are pregnant women advised not to eat liver?
5 Which mineral is found in red meat and offal such as liver?

Buying meat, poultry and offal

When you buy fresh meat, poultry or offal, make sure that it:

- is moist but not slimy or wet
- has firm, slightly springy flesh or texture
- has a good colour
- smells fresh
- has not exceeded its use-by date if it is sold in a packet.

Storing meat, poultry and meat

These foods are perishable, which means that they become unfit to eat very quickly if they are not stored correctly. If you buy them in plastic packaging, remove the packaging when you get home and place them in a covered container in the refrigerator (0 to 5°C) and use them within one to two days.

If you want to freeze fresh meat, offal or poultry, wrap it in suitable packaging to prevent exposure to the frost in the freezer (which would cause 'freezer burn' which causes foods to dry out). Place it in the 'fast freeze' compartment of the freezer to drop the temperature to at least −18°C as soon as possible.

To defrost frozen meat, offal or poultry, place the frozen product on a tray or plate (to prevent drips on to other foods) at the bottom of the refrigerator (to prevent bacterial growth as the product thaws) and allow to defrost for several hours until completely thawed.

If you want to store cooked meat, offal or poultry, allow it to cool down within 1½ hours then refrigerate or freeze. Reheat leftover cooked meat, offal or poultry once only, to avoid bacterial growth.

Did you know?

- Meat and poultry production uses up huge amounts of energy and land. About 20 times more land is used for a meat eater's diet than for a vegan's diet. Land and energy are used to grow crops to feed animals and poultry and to house them.
- Large areas of rain forest have been destroyed to produce meat.
- Most people eat more meat than they actually need.

ACTIVITY

Explain how you could make sure that the following meat-based recipes fit the Eatwell Plate and dietary guidelines, by suggesting how you might change them. For example, which ingredients you could add to them (or reduce), whether you would change the cooking method and foods you could serve with them in a meal.

- Minced beef Bolognese sauce
- Beef stew
- Grilled chicken joints
- Fried pork sausages
- Roasted lamb
- Grilled gammon steaks
- Fried pork chops
- Stir-fried chicken breasts
- Cold cooked ham
- Fried turkey steaks
- Grilled beef steaks

4.2 FISH AND SEAFOOD

WHAT ARE FISH AND SEAFOOD?

Fish and seafood are an important part of the diet for people in many countries. They are either caught from the sea or freshwater rivers and lakes or they are specially reared in large numbers on fish farms where they are held in cages.

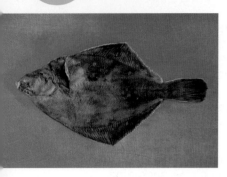

Plaice

Fish and seafood are very perishable foods and they will go 'off' and can become unsafe to eat in a few hours if they are not processed and preserved quickly after being caught. Commercial fishing boats that catch fish from the sea are like big factories where the caught fish are processed and preserved (usually by freezing) before the ship returns to the land.

Fish are either sold and eaten whole or they are cut into fillets (from flat or round fish), or as thick slices or steaks – sometimes called darnes (from round fish).

NUTRITIONAL VALUE

Fish and seafood provide the following nutrients:

- **Protein:** Fish and shellfish provide an important source of high biological value protein that is easily digested (especially white fish).
- **Fat:** Fish and shellfish both provide fat in the form of unsaturated oils. Oily fish in particular provide the essential fatty acids omega 3 and omega 6, which are known to help reduce the risk of heart disease and strokes by helping to prevent the development of blood clots.
- **Fat soluble vitamins A and D:** Oily fish are good sources of these. In white fish, the liver oils contain these vitamins and the oil is usually sold as capsules as a vitamin supplement, such as cod liver oil.
- **Group B vitamins:** Fish and shellfish both contain some B vitamins.
- **Calcium:** This is found in the bones of fish and if they are eaten (in canned fish) then they provide a useful source.
- **Fluoride and iodine**: Sea fish provide useful amounts of these and other minerals and trace elements such as sodium and potassium, but not iron.
- **Water**: Fish and seafood naturally contain water, and sometimes extra water is added to them by food processors.

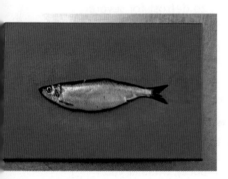

Herring

Fish and shellfish can be cooked by a variety of methods, including steaming, stir-frying, shallow and deep frying, poaching, baking and grilling. Cooking fish makes it easy to digest, and it takes little time to cook (see page 198).

TYPES OF FISH AND SEAFOOD

There are many different types of fish and seafood. Some fish is smoked over burning wood to preserve it and give it a particular flavour (kippers are smoked herrings).

The chart opposite describes some of the fish and seafood eaten in the UK.

Buying fish and shellfish

When you buy fresh fish, make sure that it:

- has firm flesh
- has moist (not slimy) skin
- is not losing lots of its scales
- has clear, shiny eyes
- has bright red gills
- has a fresh, clean smell.

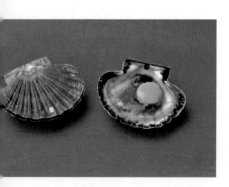

Scallops

When you buy crustaceans, make sure that they:

- smell fresh and 'sweet'
- are moist
- have no missing joints or limbs
- have firm, springy flesh (raw prawns).

When you buy molluscs, make sure that they:

- have tightly shut shells or shells that shut immediately you tap them
- smell fresh.

Type of fish/seafood	Description	Examples
White fish	Has firm white flesh Has oil in the liver, not the flesh	Flat white seawater fish: Plaice, sole, halibut
		Round white seawater fish: Cod, coley, haddock, sea bass, whiting, monkfish, hake, hoki, huss, ling, pollock, red snapper, tilapia
Oily fish	Has oil in the flesh which is quite dark	Anchovy, eel, herring, jackfish, kipper, mackerel, pilchard, salmon, sardine, sprat, swordfish, trout, tuna, whitebait
Shellfish: Molluscs	Soft-bodied sea animals that live inside shells	Cockles, winkles, mussels, scallops, clams, oysters
		Squid and cuttlefish are also in this group although they do not have shells
Crustaceans	Jointed sea animals with soft bodies covered by a hard outer skeleton or 'crust'	Lobsters, shrimps, prawns, crabs, crayfish, langoustines

ACTIVITY

1 Name two examples of white fish.
2 Name two examples of oily fish.
3 Name two examples of shellfish.
4 Which type of fish contains omega 3 fatty acids?
5 Why are these fatty acids important for our health?
6 It is recommended that we eat at least two portions of oily fish per week. Suggest two recipes that include oily fish.

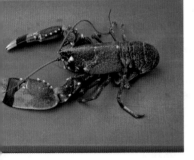

Lobster

Storing fish and shellfish

Fish and shellfish are perishable foods. That means that if they are bought fresh, they must be refrigerated and used as soon as possible – preferably on the same day. Sometimes fresh fish sold in a supermarket has been previously frozen, so it must not be refrozen.

Fresh fish can be frozen on the day that it is purchased but it must be properly wrapped to protect it from the frost in the freezer. It should be defrosted thoroughly before use.

Did you know?

- In the past sea fish were caught by people in amounts that allowed the fish to replace their numbers so that there was never a shortage of fish. But in the last few decades, the numbers of fish have decreased dramatically.
- In a lot of countries fish farming enables people to buy fish more cheaply but it can cause problems such as pollution and disease.

4.3 EGGS

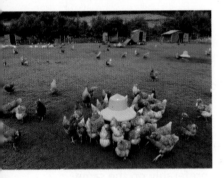

Battery farming

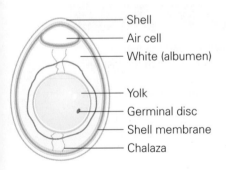

Free range hens

Inside an egg diagram

- Shell
- Air cell
- White (albumen)
- Yolk
- Germinal disc
- Shell membrane
- Chalaza

Inside an egg

Source: based on NutriPlus,
www.nutriplus.com/my

TYPES OF EGGS

In the UK we eat eggs from hens, ducks, geese and quails. The majority of eggs that we eat are from hens. If the conditions are right hens will lay eggs every day. They are then collected, graded according to their size and then packed and sold.

In the UK about 10,500 million eggs are eaten every year, and many come from battery farms where hens are kept permanently inside sheds in small cages, which are stacked on top of each other. As the hens lay the eggs, they are collected from a conveyor belt.

Hens naturally like to walk around outside, scratch the soil and peck the ground for food, lay their eggs in nests and sit up on perches at night. This is called free range egg production, and many people prefer to buy free range eggs because it is more natural. There has been an increase in the number of free range egg farms.

Some farmers keep their hens in barns so that they can walk around and peck the ground. They are not kept in cages and are provided with places to perch. This is called barn or perchery egg production.

NUTRITIONAL VALUE OF EGGS

Eggs are designed by nature to provide a place to grow a baby bird (chick), so they contain lots of different nutrients for this purpose. When you buy eggs from the shop, they are unfertilised and will not grow into a chick, but they still contain all the nutrients and so are a very useful part of our diet.

Eggs are used for a variety of functions in cooking (see page 181) and are easy to cook in a variety of ways.

Eggs give us these nutrients:
- **Protein**: in the egg white and the yolk.
- **Vitamins**: especially vitamins A, D and E in the yolk, and B vitamins (especially B_2 and B_{12}) in the white and yolk.
- **Minerals** and **trace elements**: especially phosphorus, iron (egg yolk), zinc and selenium. Calcium and other minerals are found in the shell, so we do not benefit from them.
- **Fat**: found in the yolk.
- **Water**: the egg white and yolk both contain water.
- **Energy**: a medium-sized egg provides about 80kcals (336kJ).

WHAT IS INSIDE AN EGG?

All eggs look the same inside. The table on the next page explains the different parts.

Buying eggs

Eggs are sold in four sizes:
- Very large – these weigh 73g or more.
- Large – these weigh between 63g and 73g.
- Medium – these weigh between 53g and 63g.
- Small – these weigh 53g or less.

Part of egg	What it is and what it does
Air cell (sometimes called air sac)	It forms after the egg is laid as it cools down. Fresh eggs have small air cells and the egg will sink to the bottom of a jug of salty water. Older eggs have large air cells and will float in a jug of salty water.
White – albumen	Part of this is thick and part is thin. The thick part protects the yolk. Older eggs have a larger amount of thin egg white.
Yolk	This is the centre part of the egg where the chick would grow if the egg was fertilised. The colour varies from light to darker yellow depending on what the hen has had to eat.
Germinal disc	This is where a chick would start to grow if the egg was fertilised – it contains the 'information' to make the chick.
Shell membrane	There are two of these and they help to hold the contents of the egg in place and prevent harmful bacteria from entering the egg.
Chalazae (2)	The chalazae make sure that the yolk always stays in the centre of the egg. They are made of protein.
Shell	This is the protective coating of an egg. It is covered in tiny holes (called pores) which let gases and water pass through the shell.

Did you know?

You can also buy ostrich and emu eggs in some shops. They are very large compared to hen's eggs!

ACTIVITY

1 Identify (list) three types of eggs that are eaten in the UK.
2 Which vitamins are found in the egg yolk?
3 Which vitamins are found in the egg white?
4 Which two macronutrients are found in eggs?
5 What affects the colour of the egg yolk?
6 What is the function of the shell membrane in an egg?

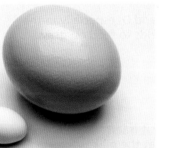

An ostrich egg shown next to a hen's egg

Storing eggs

Fresh eggs have a protective outer membrane covering the shell. If this is not removed by washing, the egg will keep fresh for a few weeks, although it will start to change inside and become watery in texture. Eventually, the egg will decompose and become very strong smelling.

It is best practice to refrigerate eggs, but they should be kept away from strong smells such as fish or garlic, as the shells are porous (contain tiny holes) and the eggs will pick up the smell of the other foods.

If an egg has a dirty shell, wash it just before using it for cooking and wash your hands afterwards. The use of eggs in cookery is covered on page 181.

ACTIVITY

Eggs are used in lots of different recipes for breakfast, midday meals, evening meals and packed lunches. Create a chart like the one below and suggest some egg recipes for each occasion.

Breakfast suggestions	Midday meal suggestions	Evening meal suggestions	Packed lunch suggestions

4.4   MILK

Milk is produced in the mammary glands by a group of animals called mammals to feed their young. Mammals include cows, sheep, pigs, dogs, cats and humans.

In the UK we mostly drink cow's milk, but sheep and goat's milk is also consumed. Milk is produced on dairy farms and sent to a dairy processing unit to be put into bottles or cartons and sold as liquid milk, or made into dairy products such as cheese, yogurt, butter and cream.

NUTRITIONAL VALUE OF MILK

Milk is designed by nature to be the only food that a baby mammal has for the first few weeks or months of its life. Therefore, milk contains everything that a baby mammal needs to enable it to grow, give it energy and help to build its immunity to disease.

Milk contains the following nutrients:

- **Protein**: This has a high biological value. Cow's milk has just over 3 per cent protein (human milk has just over 1 per cent).
- **Fat**: Cow's milk has about 3 to 4 per cent fat depending on the breed of cow the milk comes from. It contains saturated and unsaturated fatty acids, and the amounts of these depend on what the cow has been fed.
- **Carbohydrate**: Cow's milk has about 5 per cent lactose (human milk has about 7 per cent).
- **Minerals**: Milk contains a lot of calcium and good amounts of phosphorus, sodium and potassium. It has very little iron, but during pregnancy, a baby will build up a store of iron from its mother and use this until it is weaned on to solid foods.
- **Vitamins**: Milk contains a good amount of vitamins A and D, especially in the summer if the cows have been allowed out into the fields to feed on grass. It contains some B vitamins but little vitamin C.
- **Water:** Milk contains about 90 per cent water.

TYPES OF MILK

The fat in milk (cream) will float to the top of the milk if it is left to stand. To prevent this, a lot of milk is homogenised. This means that the milk is forced through a sieve with tiny holes in it, which breaks up the fat into tiny droplets that stay evenly throughout the milk and do not float to the surface.

It is possible to remove some of the fat from milk. This is called skimming. The milk is left to stand so that the fat (cream) floats to the top. The fat is then removed from the surface by skimming across it with a special tool.

This produces different types of milk:

- **Whole milk** has no fat removed – it has about 3.9 per cent fat.
- **Semi-skimmed milk** – this has a fat content of about 1.5 per cent, which is just under half the amount in whole milk.
- **Skimmed milk** – this has a fat content of about 0.1 per cent, so it is virtually fat-free

Heat treatment of milk

Milk will spoil (go off) very easily because it contains just the right conditions for bacteria to grow. To make it safe to drink and have a longer shelf-life, milk is heat treated to destroy harmful bacteria. There are several ways to heat treat milk:

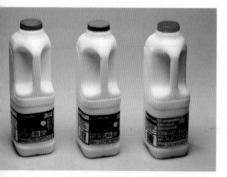

Whole, semi-skimmed and skimmed milk

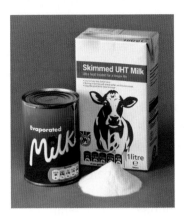

- **Pasteurisation:** This is where milk is heated very quickly to 72°C for 15 seconds and then cooled very quickly to below 10°C (usually 4°C). It is called high temperature short time (HTST) pasteurisation and takes place in a piece of machinery called a heat exchanger. The pasteurised milk must be kept in a refrigerator and used within a few days.
- **Ultra heat treated (UHT)** or **long-life:** This is where the milk is quickly heated in a heat exchanger to 132°C for one second and then rapidly cooled and packed in special sealed packs. It can be stored like this, unopened, for several months in a cupboard, but once it has been opened, it must be stored in a refrigerator and used up within a few days.
- **Dried milk:** Milk can be dried and stored in a pack then mixed with water when used.
- **Canned milk:** Milk can be heated to evaporate (reduce) some of the water it contains and kill bacteria. The evaporated milk is sealed in cans and heated again to sterilise it. Condensed milk is also evaporated and canned but has sugar added to it.

Milk for vegetarians or people with allergies

Some people do not eat any animal products, and so do not drink milk. Others are allergic to milk from mammals. For these people, it is possible to buy plant 'milks' – soya, oat, rice and coconut milks and products made from them, such as flavoured drinks. Some of these products are enriched with vitamins and minerals. Most can be used in place of milk for many recipes.

PRACTICAL ACTIVITY

Some children and teenagers do not want to drink milk but still need the nutrients that milk provides. Suggest some interesting ways in which milk could be included in their diet, other than as a drink.

Plan and make two dishes to illustrate this, giving reasons for your choice. Support your work with nutritional data.

ASSESSMENT FOR LEARNING

Look at the statements below and put a tick ✓ against all the ones you can do. If you can tick them all, well done! Make sure you can remember them in case you are asked to repeat them.

I can...

☐ Explain why milk is so important for baby mammals

☐ Describe how milk is heat treated to make it safe to drink

☐ Name three products made from milk

☐ Identify three types of fresh pasteurised cow's milk

☐ Explain why cow's milk has to be modified to make it suitable for human babies

☐ Identify which nutrients are found in milk

4.5 DAIRY PRODUCTS

Milk can be made into a range of products which add variety to the diet and are a way of preserving the milk.

CHEESE

Types of cheese

Cheese is made from the milk of cows, sheep, goats and buffalo. Whole, semi-skimmed or skimmed milk can be used to make cheese. There are hundreds of different types of cheeses, and many countries have developed their own traditional favourites.

The chart below shows the main types of cheeses, with a few examples of each.

Type of cheese	Examples
Soft cheeses: Fresh	Cream cheese, cottage cheese, quark, curd cheese, Boursin, Le Roulé, fromage frais, mascarpone, mozzarella, feta, halloumi
Ripened	Camembert, Brie, goat's, Somerset brie
Blue veined cheese (these have a special edible mould added that gives a distinct flavour and blue-coloured 'veins' through the cheese)	Blue stilton, Danish blue, Blue Wensleydale, Cambazola
Semi-soft cheeses	Stilton, gorgonzola, Wensleydale, Lancashire, Caerphilly, Edam, Raclette, St Paulin, Bel Paese, Monterey Jack
Hard cheeses	Cheddar, Gruyere, Derby, Cheshire, Double Gloucester, Leicester, Emmental, Gouda
Very hard cheese	Parmesan (parmigiano reggiano)
Whey cheeses (made from the whey with additional ingredients such as milk)	Ricotta
Processed cheese (made by mixing pieces of other cheeses together with colouring	Cheese slices, cheese spreads and flavouring)

ACTIVITY

Identify the countries each of these cheeses originally comes from.
- Camembert
- Gorgonzola
- Gouda
- Parmesan
- Gruyere
- Feta
- Caerphilly
- Wensleydale
- Monterey Jack

How cheese is made

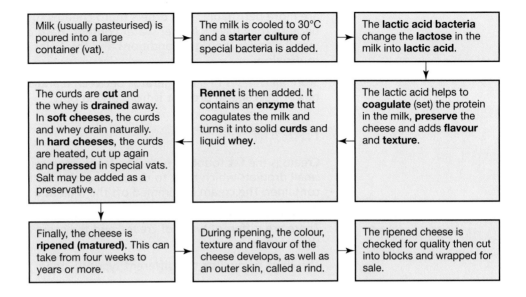

Milk (usually pasteurised) is poured into a large container (vat). → The milk is cooled to 30°C and a **starter culture** of special bacteria is added. → The **lactic acid bacteria** change the **lactose** in the milk into **lactic acid**.

The curds are **cut** and the whey is **drained** away. In **soft cheeses**, the curds and whey drain naturally. In **hard cheeses**, the curds are heated, cut up again and **pressed** in special vats. Salt may be added as a preservative. ← **Rennet** is then added. It contains an **enzyme** that coagulates the milk and turns it into solid **curds** and liquid **whey**. ← The lactic acid helps to **coagulate** (set) the protein in the milk, **preserve** the cheese and adds **flavour** and **texture**.

Finally, the cheese is **ripened (matured)**. This can take from four weeks to years or more. → During ripening, the colour, texture and flavour of the cheese develops, as well as an outer skin, called a rind. → The ripened cheese is checked for quality then cut into blocks and wrapped for sale.

Nutritional value

The amount of fat, protein and minerals varies between different types of cheeses due to the way they are processed or the milk they are made from.

Cheeses provide the following nutrients:

- **Protein:** Cheeses provide a good source of high biological value protein which is easily digested by most people. Hard cheeses have more protein than softer cheeses because they are more concentrated.
- **Fat:** Hard cheeses are about 33 per cent fat, and some full fat cream cheeses can have nearly 50 per cent fat. Soft cheeses, such as cottage cheese, have about 4 per cent fat. The fat content depends on the type of milk that was used to make the cheese. It is possible to buy reduced fat versions of many cheeses.
- **Vitamins**: Cheese is a good source of vitamin A and provides some vitamin D. It also provides some B vitamins. The amounts of vitamins vary according to what the animal that provided the milk was fed on, the time of year and how it is processed.
- **Minerals and trace elements**: Cheese is a good source of calcium, phosphorus and sodium (salt is often added as a preservative). The amounts of minerals and trace elements vary for the same reasons as for vitamins.
- **Water**: Hard cheeses provide some water (about 33 per cent), but soft cheeses contain much more (cottage cheese may contain about 80 per cent).

ACTIVITY

1 Name the main mineral found in cheese.
2 What type of protein does cheese provide?
3 Name two hard cheeses and two soft cheeses.
4 What type of bacteria change milk into cheese?

Buying cheese

Cheeses will remain fresh for several days, providing they are stored correctly. If buying pre-packed cheese, make sure that the plastic packaging is not broken anywhere as this will mean that bacteria and moulds may have got into the package.

Storing cheese

Cheese is perishable, but some types (the soft cheeses such as cottage cheese) are more perishable than others (hard cheeses such as cheddar and parmesan) because they have a higher water content. Hard cheeses can be stored for months under the right conditions and this helps their flavours and textures to develop.

Store all cheeses in a refrigerator between 0 and 5°C. Keep the cheese in a sealed box or package to prevent it from drying out.

CREAM

Cream is the fat found in milk. The fat is often called 'butterfat'. The fat is in small droplets which float to the surface of the milk when it is left to stand in a container. The cream is skimmed off the milk at a temperature of 35°C to 54°C and then it is cooled rapidly to 4°C.

There are different types of cream, and they vary according to the amount of fat they contain.

The chart below lists the different types of cream that can be bought.

Name of cream	Amount of fat it contains (In law, this is the minimum amount it should contain to be allowed to be given this name)	What it is used for
Double cream (sometimes called 'heavy' cream)	48%	Whipping, decorating (piping) desserts and cakes, pouring over food, adding to soups and sauces, adding to stews, filling pastry cases and buns, making ice cream.
Whipping cream	38%	Can be whipped up and traps air, so it has a good volume for decorating and serving with desserts and cakes.
Single cream (sometimes called 'light' cream)	18%	For pouring, adding to sauces and soups. Cannot be whipped because it does not contain enough fat.
Soured cream (treated with lactic acid which makes it slightly tangy)	20% (it is possible to buy reduced fat versions)	For dips, sauces, adding to soups, cheesecakes, jacket potato toppings, salad dressings.
Crème fraiche (similar to soured cream but milder)	35% (it is possible to buy reduced fat versions)	For desserts, dips, cheesecakes, adding to sauces, casseroles and soups. Cannot be whipped.
Clotted cream (often made from the milk of Guernsey or Jersey cows)	55%	Traditionally served with scones and jam for a 'cream tea'. Often served with desserts.
Ready 'whipped' cream (has sugar and stabilisers added plus a gas that turns it into a foam that will collapse after a while)	Depends on type	Sold in aerosols and heat-treated to have a longer shelf-life than fresh cream. Used to decorate desserts and cakes.

Nutritional value of cream

Cream provides the following nutrients:

- **Protein**: A small amount of protein is provided.
- **Fat:** The amount varies according to the cream (see chart above). The fat is mostly saturated.
- **Vitamins:** Some vitamin A and D are provided, depending on the time of year and the diet of the animal it came from. It also provides small amounts of B vitamins.
- **Minerals and trace elements:** It contains some calcium and other minerals and trace elements, depending on where the milk came from and what the animal was fed.
- **Water**: Some water is provided.

ACTIVITY

1 What is the main macronutrient in cream?
2 What is the fat content of single cream?
3 What is the fat content of double cream?
4 What is the fat content of whipping cream?

Storing cream

Cream is very perishable and so it must be stored in the refrigerator and used up within a few days. Once it is opened, cover the remaining cream in the refrigerator as it will pick up the smell of other foods.

BUTTER

Butter is made from cream. it is a natural product and has a very good flavour which is why it is often favoured by chefs and cooks in recipes instead of margarine. It can be made from any type of milk.

NUTRITIONAL VALUE OF BUTTER

Butter provides the following nutrients:

- **Protein:** It contains only a very small amount.
- **Fat:** Butter is mostly fat, much of which is saturated.
- **Vitamins:** Butter provides a good amount of vitamin A and D, depending on the time of year and the diet of the animal it came from. Butter produced from cows which have grazed on grass in the summer tends to have more than butter produced in the winter when the cows are indoors and do not have fresh grass to eat.
- **Minerals and trace elements:** It contains some minerals and trace elements, especially sodium in salted butter.
- **Water:** It contains only a small amount of water.

Types of butter

The table on the next page shows the different types of butter available.

Storing butter

Butter can be kept in a covered dish at room temperature, providing the room is not too warm. It can then be easily spread on to bread.

Butter should be stored in a refrigerator if it is not needed for spreading.

ACTIVITY

1 What is the main macronutrient in butter?
2 Why does butter produced in summer have more vitamins A and D than butter produced in winter?
3 What is the main type of fat in butter?

Types of butter	Description
Unsalted ('sweet') butter	Mild and slightly sweet
Salted butter	Before people had refrigerators, salt was added to preserve the butter, but now it is added for flavour. It is the only added ingredient.
Clarified butter	Used in cooking. It is made by slowly melting the butter and skimming off the milk solids that rise to the surface. The melted fat remains and is used for butter sauces and shallow frying.
Ghee	Clarified butter that originated in India. It has a stronger flavour than ordinary clarified butter – usually sold in cans.
Spreadable butter	This is butter that remains soft in the refrigerator because it has had some vegetable oils added to it to keep it soft.

RESEARCH ACTIVITY

Carry out a survey in your local shop to find out what is the difference between and the same about the products in the following list:

- butter
- soft margarine
- block (hard) margarine
- low fat spread
- spreadable butter.

Think about texture, colour, flavour, nutritional value, energy value (kcals), cost and what you can use it for in cooking.

YOGURT

Yogurt is a cultured milk product. This means that the milk has had a harmless, edible bacteria culture added to it to turn it into yogurt. The bacteria ferment the natural sugar (lactose) in the milk and turn it into lactic acid. This helps to give the yogurt its tangy flavour. The lactic acid coagulates (sets) the protein in the milk so the yogurt thickens.

Yogurt is eaten in many countries, and different types of milk are used to make it. It is either eaten plain (natural) or has fruit, sugar and other flavourings added to it, such as honey, lemon and vanilla. Yogurt is also sold as yogurt drinks and used as an ingredient in many sweet and savoury recipes and food products. Natural yogurt is used in the Indian drink 'lassi'.

Yogurt makes a good accompaniment to desserts and breakfast cereals instead of cream.

Nutritional value of yogurt

Yogurt provides the following nutrients:

- **Protein**: It provides a good source of high biological value protein.
- **Fat**: The amount varies according to the yogurt. Many are low fat yogurts because they are made with skimmed milk. Some yogurt-based dessert products have cream added which increases the fat content of them.
- **Carbohydrate**: There is some lactose provided and also sucrose and fructose in flavoured yogurts.

- **Vitamins:** Some vitamin A and D provided, depending on the time of year and the diet of the animal it came from. It also provides useful amounts of B vitamins.
- **Minerals and trace elements:** It contains a good source of calcium and other minerals and trace elements, depending on where the milk came from and what the animal was fed.
- **Water:** It contains a good source of water.

Types of yogurt

Type of yogurt	Description
Set yogurt	Semi-solid – the yogurt is set in the pot it is bought in. Can be natural or flavoured.
Stirred yogurt	This varies in thickness and can be poured out of the pot. Can be natural or flavoured.
Natural (plain) yogurt	Smooth, creamy texture, with a fresh, tangy flavour.
Greek (strained) yogurt	Made from cow's or ewe's (female sheep) milk. Has a high fat content and mild flavour.
Live yogurt	The bacteria in these types of yogurt are still living.

ACTIVITY

1 Which mineral is provided by yogurt?
2 Which is the main macronutrient provided by yogurt?
3 What is the main carbohydrate provided in flavoured yogurts?
4 Identify (list) four types of yogurt.

Buying yogurt

Make sure that the yogurt is within its use-by date which will be printed on the packaging.

Make sure that the lid of the yogurt has not 'blown'. If it has, it may mean that the yogurt is contaminated with yeast which has fermented the sugar inside and produced carbon dioxide gas which has caused the lid to bulge and become tight.

Storing yogurt

Store yogurt in the refrigerator and use within the use-by date.

4.6 FRUITS AND VEGETABLES

NUTRITIONAL VALUE

Green plants grow in soil and make carbohydrates using water from the soil, carbon dioxide gas from the air and energy from sunlight during a process called photosynthesis (see page 46).

Plants take up minerals from the soil through their roots and use them to grow. If the soil is rich in minerals, the plants (and us) will benefit from these.

Fruits and vegetables contain a good range of nutrients:

- **Carbohydrate:** As natural sugars, starch and fibre.
- **Vitamins:** Especially vitamin C, vitamin A (as beta carotene), and some B vitamins and vitamin E.

- **Protein**: Especially in beans, peas and lentils.
- **Minerals**: This depends on where the plant grows.
- **A variety of trace elements**: This depends on where the plant grows too.
- **Fat**: There is a little in legumes, and more in avocados, nuts and sweetcorn. Many types of nuts and corn are used to make cooking oils.
- **Water**: Fruits and vegetables are a very important source of water.
- **Fibre**: They are a very good source of fibre.

Plants also contain a wide variety of other natural substances that give them colour, flavour and texture, and that are known to be beneficial to our health, such as antioxidants.

Fruits and vegetables are therefore a very important part of our diet and we are advised to eat at least five portions a day (see page 68).

WHAT ARE FRUITS AND VEGETABLES?

Fruits and vegetables are the edible parts of plants.

There are different types of fruits:

- **Soft berry fruits** – raspberries, strawberries, blackberries, blueberries, gooseberries, bilberries and cranberries.
- **Currants** – blackcurrants, redcurrants and whitecurrants.
- **Hard fruits** – apples, pears and quinces.
- **Stone fruits** – plums, damsons, greengages, nectarines, peaches, apricots and cherries.
- **Citrus fruits** – oranges, lemons, limes, grapefruits, kumquats, tangerines, satsumas, clementines, mandarins, minneolas, ugli fruit and pomelos.
- **Exotic fruits** – bananas, star fruit (carambolas), dates, dragon fruit, passion fruit, guavas, jackfruit, kiwi fruit, mangoes, melons, lychees, sharon fruit (persimmons), physalis, pineapples, pomegranates, figs and grapes.

Vegetables are the other parts of plants and include:

- **Roots** – carrots, beetroot, parsnips, radishes, celeriac, swede and turnip.
- **Tubers** (found under the ground attached to roots) – potatoes, sweet potatoes and Jerusalem artichokes.
- **Bulbs** – onions, leeks, spring onions, chives, shallots and garlic.
- **Stems** – asparagus, celery, rhubarb, fennel, chicory and asparagus.
- **Leaves** – cabbage, lettuce, Brussels sprouts, kale, watercress, spinach and pak choi.
- **Flower heads** – cauliflower, broccoli (calabrese) and globe artichokes.
- **Fungi** – flat, chestnut and button mushrooms.

Some fruits we use as vegetables, such as tomatoes, avocado pears, okra, peppers (capsicums), aubergines, olives, cucumbers, sweetcorn, marrows, butternut squashes and courgettes.

Beans (runner, broad, kidney, soya, French, borlotti and haricot), peas (green peas, chick peas, split peas) and lentils (orange, brown and green puy) are really seeds, but we use them as vegetables. In some cases, they are eaten on their own and in others they are eaten with the pods they grow in. They are given the general name of legumes.

Beans can be sprouted to produce tender, juicy bean sprouts which are either eaten raw or added to stir fries. They contain a rich source of vitamin C.

Nuts are also the fruits of plants.

How do we use fruits?

There are many ways we can eat fruit:

- They can either be eaten raw, with or without their skins and seeds.
- They can be stewed in water to soften them.

ACTIVITY

Design a leaflet to encourage teenagers to eat '5-a-day'. Include a recipe suggestion on the back of your leaflet.

- They can be baked in the oven – apples and plums.
- Some fruits are fried as fritters – pineapple, banana and apple.
- A number of fruits can be dried. Grapes can be dried to produce sultanas, raisins or currants; bananas can be made into banana chips; and plums can be dried to produce prunes.
- Some fruits freeze well, such as raspberries and blackberries. Others can be pureed then frozen on their own or in ice creams and sorbets.
- Some fruits are canned, bottled in syrup or preserved as jams or chutneys.
- Some fruits can be preserved in sugar (called 'crystallised' or 'candied' fruits) – cherries, lemon and orange peel, pineapple.
- Fruits can be blended to produce smoothie drinks and fruit sauces (called 'coulis' (pronounced 'coo – lee').
- Fresh fruits can be added to jellies and mousses, except for pineapple and kiwi fruits which contain substances that stop jelly and mousses made with gelatine from setting.
- Fruits are added to some savoury dishes – apple with pork, lemon with chicken, mangoes in curry, cranberries in meat pies, grapes with fish.

How do we use vegetables?

There are also many ways we can eat vegetables:

- Some vegetables are eaten raw, with or without their skins, in salads and as side dishes for some recipes such as curries.
- Vegetables can be made into a wide range of soups and are used to flavour stocks made from meat or fish bones or sauces.
- Vegetables can be roasted, baked, fried, stir-fried, grilled, barbequed, boiled, steamed, stewed and braised and cooked in the microwave oven.
- Many vegetables are canned, but the heat involved in this process can damage their texture, colour and nutritional value.
- Some vegetables are dried – onions, tomatoes.
- Some vegetables are preserved in vinegar – onions, cucumbers, chutneys and pickles.
- Vegetables are usually served as accompaniments to other foods in a meal, but they are also used as the main part of a meal in many recipes such as vegetable curries, pies, flans, risottos, pasta meals, in a cheese sauce, or as containers for other ingredients (stuffed peppers, stuffed courgettes, jacket potatoes).

Many vegetables are frozen, which often helps to preserve their nutritional value. Very watery vegetables such as cucumbers do not freeze very well and become very soft when they are defrosted.

Buying fruits and vegetables

It is best to eat fruits and vegetables when they have just been picked or dug up as this is when they have the most nutrients in them. But this is not always possible, as when you buy them from the supermarket or shop, they may already be several days old. This means that you need to store them in a cool, dark place and use them up as quickly as possible.

Always try to choose fruits and vegetables that are not bruised, mouldy, damaged or soft and wilted.

Storing fruits and vegetables

Wash fruits and vegetables before using them to remove soil, dust, insects and some pesticide sprays.

Store salad and green vegetables in the refrigerator in a box to keep them fresh.

Use fruits and vegetables within a few days of purchase when they will be at their freshest and most nutritious. Use bruised or damaged fruits and vegetables first. Remove any bruised or damaged fruits from the fruit bowl as they will quickly become mouldy and cause others to be the same.

PRACTICAL ACTIVITY

Imagine you are deciding what to make for your evening meal and want to use up the following ingredients that you have in your refrigerator:

- 4 spring onions
- Half a red pepper
- Half a yellow pepper
- ½ a bulb of garlic
- A handful of spinach
- 3 mushrooms
- Some leftover roasted sweet potato
- Some stewed apple
- A few strawberries that are starting to go soft.

Work out an interesting and tasty meal that includes these ingredients (you can add other ingredients that you would have in the store cupboard).

ACTIVITY

The photo below shows a variety of fruits.

Here are the names of these fruits. Match the name of each with the photograph.

banana	pear	peach	pineapple
water melon	plum	cherry	orange

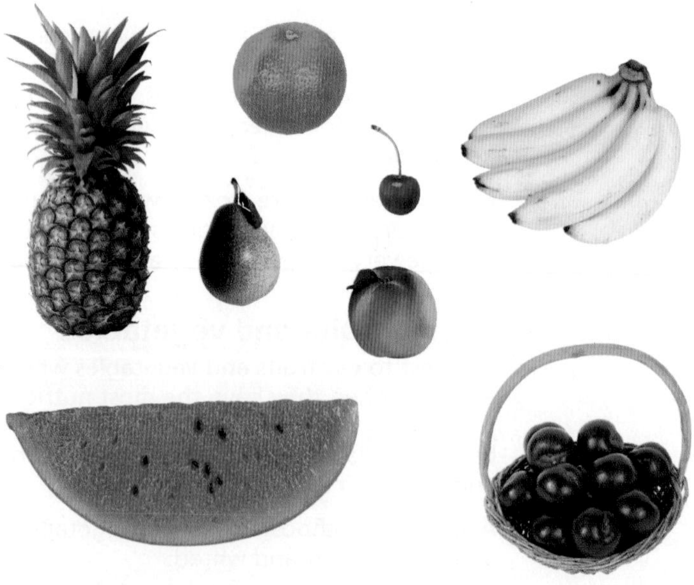

CEREALS AND CEREAL PRODUCTS

WHAT ARE CEREALS?

Cereals are the grains (seeds) of plants, most of which are types of cultivated grass. Cereal grains have been the most important (staple) foods of many countries for thousands of years. The climate and type of soil affects which cereals are grown and how important they are in a country or area of a country.

They provide people with the main source of energy in their diets and they can be made into a wide variety of food products.

NUTRITIONAL VALUE OF CEREALS

Plants produce seeds at the end of their growing season to enable new plants to grow the following year. Seeds therefore contain all the nutrients needed for a new plant to grow, so they are very nutritious for us too.

The best way to get all the nutrients from cereal seeds is to eat the whole seed – we call these unrefined or wholegrain/wholemeal cereals. Unrefined, wholegrain cereals give us these nutrients:

- protein
- carbohydrate (especially starch)
- group B vitamins
- fat (a little)
- iron
- vitamin E
- a variety of trace elements
- a very good source of fibre.

Types of cereals
The chart below tells you:

- what they are used for
- whether or not they contain gluten (which you would need to know if you have coeliac disease which means that your body cannot tolerate gluten and it prevents you from absorbing some other nutrients).

Type of cereal	What it is used for	Contains gluten?
Barley	<ul><li>Animal feed</li><li>Making beer and whisky</li><li>Can be made into bread</li><li>Pearl barley used in soups and stews</li><li>Barley flakes used in breakfast cereals</li><li>Can be cooked on its own as an alternative to rice</li><li>Malt extract is obtained from barley – used as a sweetener in foods (maltose)</li></ul>	Yes
Buckwheat	<ul><li>Not a cereal grass, but the seeds are used to make flour or eaten like rice</li><li>Used to make buckwheat pasta</li><li>Very nutritious – very good source of calcium</li></ul>	No

Type of cereal	What it is used for	Contains gluten?
Corn (maize)	• Used for human and animal food and to produce a variety of products, e.g. corn oil, high fructose corn syrup (used to sweeten fizzy drinks) and cornflour (corn starch is used to thicken foods such as custard) • Cornmeal (polenta) is used to make breads, cakes, biscuits, pancakes, tortillas, muffins and fried snack foods • Fresh maize (corn on the cob) is eaten as a vegetable • Dried maize is used for popcorn	No
Millet	• A good source of iron • It can be used as an alternative to rice but the seeds have to be heated first to make them crack so that they will take up water and become soft • Millet flakes are added to breakfast cereals or used for porridge	No
Oats	• Very nutritious and cheap to buy – provides a good amount of calcium • Available as oatmeal, porridge oats or jumbo oat flakes • Used for porridge • Added to breads, cakes, biscuits and fruit crumble toppings • Made into oatcakes, flapjacks and oat crackers	A little (but not enough to make bread)
Quinoa (this is how you say it: 'keen-wah')	• Not a type of grass but the seeds are used as an alternative to rice • Very nutritious – contains a lot of protein (but not gluten)	No
Rice	• Grown in many parts of the world – a very important cereal as it provides a lot of energy and B vitamins • There are many varieties and some of them have long grains and some have short, round grains • Long grain rice is used traditionally for savoury dishes (e.g. basmati, patna, easy-cook, brown wholegrain) • Short grain rice is used traditionally for sweet dishes (e.g. pudding rice) • Speciality rice, e.g. Arborio risotto, Thai fragrant rice • Rice flour is used for desserts, to add texture to biscuits, cakes and pancakes • Rice flakes can be made into porridge	No
Rye	• Used to make bread • Kibbled rye (seeds which have been broken up) is added to granary bread • Rye flakes are added to breakfast cereals	Yes, but not as much as wheat, so rye bread is much denser in texture. You can mix rye with wheat flour to make lighter bread
Spelt	• Similar to wheat but has more protein • Used for bread making, pasta and other baked goods	The protein has a different structure than ordinary wheat so it can be eaten by some people who have a wheat allergy or intolerance

▶

Type of cereal	What it is used for	Contains gluten?
Wheat	• Very important cereal in many parts of the world • Used in all types of baked products, e.g. breads, pastries, cakes, biscuits, puddings • Whole grains can be cooked and served like rice and can be cracked and kibbled • Bulgur wheat is steamed whole grains, which are then cracked and soaked in boiling water before eating • Couscous is steamed, dried and cracked grains of durum wheat (a variety of wheat that is used to make pasta), often used as an alternative to boiled rice • Wheat flakes are used in breakfast cereals • Wheat bran can be bought and added to recipes • Wheat germ contains a lot of vitamin E and other nutrients and can be added to recipes like wheat bran • Other products are made from milling the wheat, e.g. semolina, which is used in puddings and for adding texture to cakes and biscuits	Yes

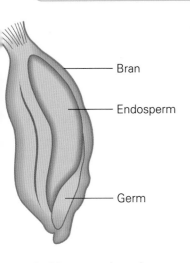

Inside a cereal seed

Inside the seed

All cereal seeds look similar inside. The diagram shows you a simple plan of what they look like:

The outer layers of the seed are known as the bran. This is where most of the fibre is found, plus many of the vitamins, minerals and trace elements as well as some of the protein and fat.

The middle (main) part of the seed is called the endosperm. This where the carbohydrate (starch) and most of the protein is found, plus some of the vitamins.

The smallest part of the seed is called the germ (this is not the same as the word we use for something that causes a disease). This contains the new shoot and the 'information' the seed will need to grow into a new plant when the seed germinates. It contains most of the fat, some of the protein and vitamins, minerals and trace elements.

Processing cereal grains

Many cereals are processed before we eat them. The most common process is milling to make flour. The seeds are broken down by millstones (this is what most windmills or water mills were used for) or metal rollers in a modern factory. The milled flour can be sieved to remove different parts of the seeds:

White wheat flour has about 30 per cent of the seed removed (the bran and germ) and therefore contains 70 per cent of the seed. Wholemeal wheat flour has none of the seed removed and therefore contains 100 per cent of the seed.

Other types of cereal seeds are processed to remove the tough outer layers (sometimes called the 'husk') of the seeds. Rice is 'polished', barley is 'pearled' and oats are 'hulled'.

If parts of the seeds are removed, this means that some of the nutrients are lost as well. Therefore it is best to eat wholegrain seeds and their products to get all of the nutrients.

Bread making

Most countries have traditional breads, which are made from cereal flour. Breads provide a nutritious and filling food, which can be eaten at any time of the day with other foods as part of a meal or as a 'container' for other foods (sandwiches, wraps, tortillas, pittas).

Breads are either unleavened (flat, unrisen) or leavened (risen, usually with yeast). To make leavened bread rise, the protein called gluten needs to be present in the cereal flour. Gluten absorbs water as the bread dough is made and makes the dough very stretchy so that it will rise when the yeast starts to produce carbon dioxide gas bubbles. Flour with a high gluten content is needed to make bread, choux and puff pastry. This is called strong plain bread flour.

To make cakes, biscuits and other pastries that do not need to rise so much, flour with a lower gluten content is used. This is called soft plain flour. This can be made into self raising flour by adding baking powder to it.

Some people suffer from gluten intolerance (coeliac disease, see page 149), which means that they must avoid any foods that contain gluten.

Other uses of cereals

Whole grains can be added to casseroles, soups and stews or boiled until soft and served with a meal.

Cracked or 'kibbled' grains (kibbled wheat and bulgur wheat) are cut or broken pieces of whole grains that can be added to breads, biscuits, soups, stews etc.

'Meal', which is a type of coarse flour, can be made into porridge (corn meal, oat meal) or used to thicken soups and stews.

Many types of cereal grains are processed into breakfast cereals, by heat treating them (toasting, puffing, flaking) and adding flavourings such as different sugars, colours and other ingredients such as chocolate powder, dried fruit, extra bran or honey.

PRACTICAL ACTIVITY

Plan and make a dish suitable for someone with coeliac disease.

Give reasons for your choice of ingredients.

4.8 SUGARS AND SWEETNERS

WHAT IS SUGAR?

Sugar has been added to foods and drinks for many centuries as a flavouring and a preservative. It is used in a wide range of recipes to provide colour, texture, flavour and, in some cases, to trap air to make a mixture light.

Most people like foods and drinks with a sweet taste, but we know that a high consumption of sugars can be damaging to our health, because it can lead to obesity and tooth decay. So current dietary guidelines recommend that we eat only a small amount of added sugar in our diet.

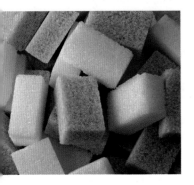

Brown and white lump sugar

NUTRITIONAL VALUE OF SUGARS AND SWEETENERS

Sugars and sweeteners provide the following nutrients:

- **Carbohydrate**: Natural refined sugars such as sucrose are virtually 100 per cent carbohydrate.
- **Minerals and trace elements:** Some of the brown sugars and syrups that contain molasses have some minerals and trace elements, such as iron and calcium, but the amount varies according to how they have been processed. Honeys contain varying amounts of iron, copper, calcium, potassium and magnesium.
- **Vitamins:** Honeys provide some B vitamins, especially thiamin, riboflavin and niacin.

Suggestions for reducing sugar in the diet

You can reduce the quantity of added sugar in recipes as most recipes will still work if the sugar content is reduced.

You can use alternative naturally sweet foods in recipes such as carrots (carrot cake), ripe fresh fruits (bananas, apples, pears, grapes, pineapple) and dried fruits (currants, sultanas, apricots, apples, papaya, mango, raisins).

You can also use food sweeteners, which add flavour but no sugar.

Types of natural sweeteners

Natural sweeteners are natural sugars made by plants and extracted from them to be added to food to sweeten it and include:

- cane sugar – this comes from the stems of a very tall grass, which is mostly grown in tropical countries

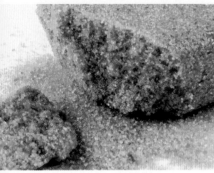

Demerara sugar

- beet sugar – this comes from the root of a plant which looks a bit like a large parsnip, and is grown mostly in northern temperate countries.

Both of these produce sucrose, which is the sugar that is used in cooking and added to many foods. During the production of sugar, crystals of sucrose are produced which give the sugar its 'sparkle' and crunchy texture. The sucrose is available in different forms as shown below.

Type of sugar (sucrose)	Description
Muscovado (molasses) sugar	Dark brown, strongly flavoured, moist and made of small, fine crystals
Demerara (raw) sugar	Light brown, contains some molasses, slightly moist and made of medium-sized crystals that make it 'crunchy'
Light, soft brown sugar	Light brown, with a 'syrupy' flavour and made of fine crystals
White granulated sugar	Refined (no molasses), all-purpose sugar with medium-sized crystals
White caster (superfine) sugar	Refined (no molasses) sugar with very small crystals
Icing (confectioner's) sugar	White (no molasses) sugar made by grinding into a fine powder; sometimes has anti-caking agent added to stop it from sticking together in lumps

Honey is also natural and is produced by honey bees from the nectar they collect from flowers. The colour, texture and flavour vary according to the flowers the bees have collected nectar from. The honey is either eaten as honeycomb straight from beehives or is heat treated and processed into clear, runny honey or sold as crystallised solid honey.

Syrups are natural sweeteners and there are several different types, as shown below.

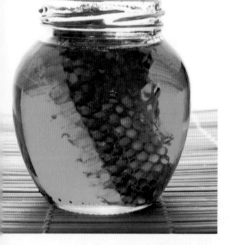

Runny honey with a piece of honeycomb

Type of syrup	Description
Maple syrup	Made from the sap (plant juices) of the maple tree, with a distinctive flavour. Sweeter than sugar
Golden syrup	Light, golden colour with a distinctive flavour. Made from cane sugar
Black treacle	Thick, black and very sticky. Made from refined molasses. Has a very strong, slightly bitter flavour
Molasses	Varies in colour and thickness – the thickest is blackstrap molasses which contains less sugar. Usually contains a range of minerals and trace elements including iron, calcium magnesium, phosphorus and zinc

Types of artificial sweeteners

Artificial sweeteners are chemical sweeteners that are made in a laboratory and sold as liquids, tablets, powders or crystals. They are much sweeter than natural sugars and so are used in tiny amounts to sweeten drinks and other foods.

Artificial sweeteners do not supply the body with energy so they are often used in low sugar or sugar-free food products and drinks aimed at people who are trying to lose weight.

There are several types:

- saccharin
- aspartame
- acesulfame k
- sucralose.

Aspartame should not be given to people who have a quite rare health condition called phenylketonuria (PKU), because it contains a substance that they cannot digest and that would make their condition worse.

ASSESSMENT FOR LEARNING

When you are making your own food, recipes often tell you to add a particular amount of sucrose (sugar). Look at the list of recipes that all tell you to add sucrose. Suggest some ways in which you could reduce the sweetness and the sucrose content of these recipes to help someone who is trying to reduce the amount of sugar in their diet.

- Custard sauce
- Fruit crumble
- Apple pie
- Chocolate cake
- Cheesecake
- Fruit scones
- Rice or sago pudding
- Baklava
- Cookies

TOPIC 5

CONVENIENCE, ORGANIC AND FUNCTIONAL FOODS

5.1 CONVENIENCE FOODS

Convenience foods are food products which are made by food manufacturers rather than at home by consumers or in a restaurant by caterers.

Convenience foods get their name because they:

- save consumers and caterers time and effort
- make the preparation of meals easier for consumers and caterers
- have a long shelf-life so that they can be stored, to save time shopping
- are sold in 'portion controlled' sizes, for example one, two or four servings, to make meal planning and preparation easier.

Who might find convenience foods very useful?

- People who have little time available to prepare and cook a meal.
- People who are physically disabled and have difficulty in preparing foods.
- Single people who are just feeding themselves.
- People with limited kitchen facilities.
- People with limited cooking skills.
- Caterers in hotels, pubs, restaurants, canteens, cafés and other places where food is provided for people – to save time and money and make their businesses more efficient.

There are lots of different convenience foods, and the chart below shows how they are divided into groups.

Group	Type of convenience food	Examples
Meals	**Complete (ready to eat) meals**	
	Cook-chill: meals which are cooked in bulk in a factory, then portioned into containers and rapidly chilled to keep them safe to eat	Curries, Chinese food, pies, flans, stews, pasta- and rice-based meals, fish meals
	Frozen and ready to cook from frozen or after defrosting	Complete roast dinners, pies, flans, vegetarian meals, cottage pie, fish pie, desserts
	Bottled	Baby foods
	Canned	Baby foods, stews, curries
	Dried	Instant noodle pot meals
	Fast foods: cooked quickly for the customer and usually eaten with the hands from the packet or wrapper	Burgers, fries, pizzas, fish and chips, fried chicken
	Take-away foods: prepared, cooked and taken away in containers to serve at home	Complete meals such as Indian and Chinese meals; sandwiches, wraps and filled rolls; snacks; hot drinks; croissants, pasties and pies; salads

Group	Type of convenience food	Examples
Parts of meals	Sauces	Pasta sauces, cheese sauce, custard, fruit, gravy
	Soups	Dried, fresh, canned, instant
	Salads	Salads in bags, e.g. mixed leaf; coleslaw; potato salad; pasta salad; bean salad; fruit salad
	Vegetables	Peeled, chopped and grated fresh vegetables; frozen; canned; bottled; potato products such as chips, waffles, roasted, mashed with flavourings
	Desserts	Frozen, e.g. cheesecakes, gateaux, flans; dried instant, e.g. fruit-flavoured 'whips' made with milk or water; fresh, e.g. flans, tortes, gateaux, pavlovas, roulades; canned, e.g. milk puddings such as rice, canned fruit, pie fillings; bottled, e.g. fruits in syrup, fruit and chocolate sauces
	Soups	Canned, dried, 'instant', fresh (cartons)
	Meat, poultry and fish	Cooked meat products such as pies and pasties, processed sliced meat, canned meat balls, canned chicken in white sauce, shaped and breaded chicken pieces for frying or baking, filleted fish coated with batter or breadcrumbs
	Other foods	Ready-made party food, frozen Yorkshire puddings, sliced bread, cereal bars, celebration cakes, fresh pasta products, packed lunch items such as breadsticks with dips, cakes, cookies and biscuits
Ingredients	Stocks for use in stews, soups, etc.	Stock cubes or fresh liquid stock in different flavours, e.g. beef, fish, chicken, vegetable
	Dried packet mixes – usually have to be mixed with other ingredients, e.g. eggs, oil, milk	Cakes, cookies and biscuits, scones, pastry, batters, vegetable burger mix, instant dessert mixes, trifle mix, bread mixes, crumble toppings
	Fresh ingredients	Pastry (puff and short crust), pizza bases, part-baked bread rolls and loaves, prepared vegetables for stir-fry meals, sandwich fillings, whipped cream in an aerosol can
	Sauces	For pasta; to cook with meat or poultry; to add to stir-fry meals; to flavour other dishes

DISADVANTAGES OF CONVENIENCE FOODS

Convenience foods tend to use a lot of packaging, which means that there are issues with their effects on the environment (disposal of used packaging) and on non-renewable resources (oil is needed to make plastics).

Many health professionals are concerned about the amounts of fat, sugar, salt and food additives that are used in convenience foods, and the effects these may have on people's health.

Using convenience foods means that people do not use their own skills to make foods 'from scratch', using fresh ingredients. This means that there has been a decline in the number of people who know how to cook.

ACTIVITY

1 What is meant by the term 'convenience food'?
2 Describe three advantages of using convenience foods.
3 Identify three groups of people who may find it useful to use convenience foods.
4 Explain why convenience foods are useful to each of the groups you have identified.
5 Give two examples of convenience food meals.
6 Give two examples of fast food convenience meals.
7 Give two examples of ingredients that are convenience foods.

EXTENSION ACTIVITY

Convenience foods are very much a part of most people's daily intake of food. Using the list of issues below as a guide, and the list of convenience foods in the chart above, list the advantages and disadvantages of convenience foods for people, the food industry and society, giving reasons for your answers.

- Cost (ingredients, compared to home made)
- Impact on the environment (production, packaging, disposal)
- Health (long and short term)
- Use of resources (time, energy, materials)
- Cooking skills

RESEARCH ACTIVITY

A youth club wants to start serving hot snacks and drinks to the club members. The cooking facilities are very limited (a small cooker and a microwave oven), but there is a reasonably sized food preparation area and space to store foods on shelves and in a refrigerator. The organisers want to produce a variety of foods to suit different food preferences and cultures.

Suggest some foods that the youth club could serve, and make a list of convenience foods they could use to make their task easier within their limited facilities.

PRACTICAL ACTIVITY

For one food, such as tomato soup, make different versions as follows:

a) all fresh ingredients, made from scratch
b) some fresh ingredients plus some canned tomatoes
c) a fresh convenience tomato soup
d) a dried convenience tomato soup
e) a canned convenience tomato soup.

Compare the different versions for:

- price
- time taken to prepare
- flavour, colour and texture
- preference (set up a tasting panel)
- nutritional value.

Evaluate your findings.

5.2 GENETICALLY MODIFIED FOODS

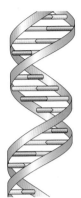

DNA

WHAT ARE GENES?

The word 'genetically' comes from the word 'gene'.

In all living organisms (plants and animals), genes control the characteristics that are passed on from one generation to the next generation. This might be colour of petals, skin colour, type of hair or fur. This is called 'genetic inheritance' – plants and animals inherit characteristics from their parents.

Genes are found in every cell of a living organism and are copied whenever a cell divides and reproduces. They are made up of a chemical substance called DNA (deoxyribonucleic acid). DNA is made up of two long strands intertwined in a spiral known as a double helix (it looks a bit like a ladder that has been twisted).

Each strand of the helix contains four amino acids which are put together in different sequences to create a code of instructions for each characteristic.

WHAT IS GENETIC MODIFICATION?

Genetic modification (GM) is a relatively new and complex branch of science.

The principle of GM is to copy a gene with its code for a particular characteristic and insert it into another living organism. This will then be able to produce that characteristic because it can follow the coded instructions.

Genetic engineers make use of specific enzymes to do this. The enzymes can 'unzip' double strands of DNA, cut the DNA at specific points, copy DNA and 'paste' sections of DNA into the gene.

GM crops

Why is GM carried out?

In the past, farmers have selected certain plants or animals with specific characteristics for growing the next season to produce better crops or offspring. A chosen plant may produce bigger seeds or deeper coloured fruit or an animal may produce bigger offspring.

GM aims to create new genetic material for farmers and breeders to work on. Genes can be transferred in ways that were not possible before.

The most commonly grown GM crops are oilseed rape, soya bean, cotton, kiwi fruit, maize, sugar beet, potato and tomato. Characteristics that have been engineered into plant crops include:

- better resistance to weed-killing chemicals (so that the weeds get killed but not the crop)
- increased storage or shelf-life
- better resistance to insects, fungi and bacteria that could affect the crop.

GM bacteria, fungi, animals and fish are also being developed for use in food production. Characteristics that have been engineered into animals include:

- faster growing rates
- less fat
- better resistance to disease.

Concerns about GM

Many people are concerned about the use of GM foods for a variety of reasons, including:

- The pollen from GM crops could escape and mix with wild plants, which would affect the ecology of an area.
- New resistant micro-organisms could develop which could cause problems in plants and animals.
- Some people may become allergic to GM foods if DNA from certain plants or animals, which are known to cause allergies, are put into others.
- Many GM crops sold by large companies have a 'terminator gene' built into them. This means that the seeds are not fertile, so farmers cannot keep some seeds to grow next year (which is a traditional practice) but have to buy a new set of seeds each year. This ties them to a GM company and they risk losing their livelihood if the GM company decides not to grow the crop any longer. This would particularly affect poor farmers in developing countries.

WHICH FOODS ARE GM?

There are a number of foods that have been genetically modified. It is not possible to tell by looking at them if they are GM or not. The only way to know is if a food manufacturer gives this information on a food label. When GM foods were first brought out, there were lots of objections and some of the supermarket companies in the UK decided they would not sell them. These foods included soya beans, sweetcorn, sugar beet and sugar cane, rapeseed, tomatoes and some types of rice.

5.3 ORGANIC FOODS

WHAT ARE ORGANIC FOODS?

Organic foods are produced using organic farming methods, in which farmers aim to produce food that is grown in well-balanced, healthy, living soil without the use of artificial chemical fertilisers and pesticides. Farmers are allowed to use about four of the many hundreds of pesticides as a last resort if they have a problem, but the use is very strictly controlled.)

Organically produced animals are reared without the routine use of medicines, in the most natural conditions possible. For example, organic chickens are allowed to live outside (free range) where they can follow their natural instincts, scratch around in the soil to find insects to eat, exercise their legs and wings, and go back into a house at night to sleep on a perch.

Organic farming

Organic farmers aim to produce food as naturally as possible and avoid unbalancing the **ecosystem** of the soil, in which millions of different tiny animals live and recycle the nutrients that come into the soil from leaves, dead plants, manure from animals, rain and so on. When plants grow in the soil, they take out a lot of nutrients, which can make the soil unbalanced if the nutrients are not replaced.

Artificial fertilisers (used in intensive farming) do not build good soil because they do not feed all the tiny animals or maintain the soil structure, and so the soil becomes less balanced.

Organic farming encourages **crop rotation**, where the farmer plants one crop, such as wheat, in a field one year, then grazes animals on the same field the following year, to add manure to the soil; in the third year, the farmer may leave the field **fallow** (without a crop or animals) to allow the soil to recover its nutrient balance and structure naturally.

Organic foods

The word 'organic' has a legal definition and organic foods have a symbol on the label to prove that they have been produced organically. In other countries, different words are used, such as 'bio', 'oko' or 'eco', which you may see on some food labels.

In the UK, a Soil Association or Organic Farmers and Growers symbol certifies that a food really is organically produced.

Most of our food is grown by modern **intensive farming**. This means that large numbers of plants or animals are produced in one place using:

- lots of **machinery**
- **artificial fertilisers** to put nutrients into the soil
- **pesticides** to kill insects, moulds and weeds which would affect the growth of a crop
- **antibiotics** and other medicines to stop diseases spreading among animals and birds
- **growth promoters** to make animals and birds grow quickly.

An example is the intensive production of chicken, in which large numbers of chickens (about 25,000 birds) are kept in large sheds which are artificially lit and heated. The chickens are given a feed that makes them grow very fast and they are slaughtered after 42 days. Many of them suffer from problems with their legs and feet, because they get very heavy and cannot run about to keep their weight down. Because the chickens live in very crowded conditions, diseases can spread very quickly.

WHY BUY ORGANIC FOODS?

Sales of organic foods have increased over the last few years. There are a variety of reasons for this, including the following:

- Many people consider that organic foods taste better because they have been grown naturally in good soil conditions.
- Many people are concerned about the pesticides that are used on non-organic foods and the effects these may have on our health.
- Many people are concerned about the effects of intensive farming on the environment and so prefer to buy foods that have been organically farmed.

Organic foods can be bought in many places in the UK.

- Most supermarkets sell a range of fresh and processed organic foods.
- There are a few supermarkets that sell only organic foods.
- Many farmer's markets sell organically produced foods.
- Organic farm shops sell food grown on the farm.
- Many companies operate organic box schemes where you pay for a box of organic fruits and vegetables to be delivered to your house or to a collection point.
- Some companies sell organic foods by mail order.

5.4   FUNCTIONAL FOODS

WHAT ARE FUNCTIONAL FOODS?

In the 1980s, health experts in Japan described how certain foods contain substances other than nutrients that can have a positive effect on health and well-being. They called these 'functional foods'.

There is no legal definition of functional foods, but they are generally described as foods that you would eat as part of a normal diet, that contain naturally occurring substances that can lower your risk of developing certain diseases and enhance your general health.

Examples of functional foods include:
- foods that contain rich sources of specific nutrients such as minerals, vitamins, fatty acids or NSP (fibre)
- foods that contain biologically active substances such as phytochemicals (see below) or other antioxidants
- foods called probiotics that contain live beneficial bacterial cultures, such as yogurts, yogurt drinks and some cheeses.

WHAT DO NATURAL FOODS CONTAIN?

Natural foods are composed of hundreds of different natural chemicals. All these natural chemicals make up the characteristics of each food: its colour(s), flavour, texture, smell, acidity and nutritional value.

Plant foods are described as functional foods because they contain many substances that it is thought can benefit (be good for) our health.

These substances are called phytochemicals ('phyto' is the Greek word for plant), and there are more than 1,000 that we know about.

There is a lot of interest and research being carried out into these substances, and health professionals suggest it is a good idea for people to eat natural foods as part of their diet every day in order to benefit from them.

Phytochemicals are not called nutrients because they are not vital for life and are not stored in the body, but we do know that many of them do important jobs in the body to help keep it healthy and working properly.

Where can phytochemicals be found?

Certain groups of plant foods are known to be particularly good sources of phytochemicals. These include:
- Onions, garlic, leeks, shallots, chives
- Naturally brightly coloured fruits and vegetables
- Citrus fruits: oranges, grapefruit, lemons, limes, clementines, satsumas
- Tomatoes
- Green leafy vegetables
- Vegetables such as broccoli, Brussels sprouts, cabbage, cauliflower, cress, horseradish, kale, kohlrabi, mustard, radishes and turnips
- Soya and soya products such as tofu, tempeh, miso and other beans and lentils
- Ginger, turmeric and other spices
- Berries such as blueberries, strawberries, blackcurrants and goji berries
- Nuts and seeds
- Certain types of tea, such as green tea
- Fresh herbs
- Wholegrain cereals.

Did you know?

The natural flavour of a raspberry is made up of at least 131 different flavour molecules!

FUNCTIONAL FOODS AND HEALTH

The chart lists some specific functional foods and the benefits to health that these foods may have, according to research.

Functional food	Suggested health benefits
Whole oat products, e.g. porridge, oat cereals, oat bran, oat biscuits	Lower blood cholesterol levels and reduce the risk of developing heart disease
Foods made from soya beans, e.g. tofu, tempeh, miso, soya milk	
Special margarines made with plant stanols and sterol esters, e.g. Benecol	
Oily fish containing omega-3 fatty acids	Reduce the risk of heart disease
Cranberry juice	Reduce the risk of urinary tract infections
Garlic	Lower blood cholesterol levels
Green tea	Reduce the risk of developing some cancers
Tomatoes and tomato products	Reduce the risk of developing some cancers, especially prostate cancer
Dark green leafy vegetables, e.g. spinach	Reduce the risk of developing serious eye illnesses that may lead to blindness
Probiotics, e.g. live yogurt	Beneficial effects on the intestines and immune system

ACTIVITY

1 What is meant by the term 'functional foods'?
2 Give two examples of functional foods.
3 Name four functional foods and describe the possible benefits to health.
4 Suggest a good breakfast for a person who is trying to reduce their blood cholesterol levels.

RESEARCH ACTIVITY

1 Dietary guidelines sometimes suggest that we should 'eat a rainbow' in order to eat well and be healthy. What do you think they mean by this?
2 Why do natural foods usually have a better nutritional value than processed foods?

ACTIVITY

1 Plan four main meals for a family of two adults and two children (aged 6 and 8 years) based on the 'eat a rainbow' dietary advice. Explain why you have chosen the foods in your menus.
2 Carry out a survey of products in your local supermarket and make a list of the products that are advertised as being rich in particular nutrients or probiotics. Which people do you think these products are targeted at? Comment on the price, the packaging and the other ingredients in the products.

TOPIC

6

A BALANCED DIET

WHAT IS A BALANCED DIET?

There is a lot of evidence to show that what we eat has a definite influence on our health and well-being. From a young age, our daily eating habits can have a direct effect on whether or not we develop diet-related health conditions such as obesity, heart disease and diabetes when we are older.

The basic principle of eating for good health is to eat a balanced diet.
A balanced diet is one that provides you with:

- a wide variety of foods that contain different nutrients
- the right amount of nutrients for your needs
- a variety of natural food textures, flavours and colours.

The Eatwell Plate (see page 67) shows the amounts of different groups of foods that we should eat to provide us with a balanced diet.

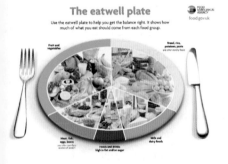

Source: Food Standards Agency

ACTIVITY

Look at how the Eatwell Plate is divided into sections. The bigger the section is, the more of those foods we should eat.

Which two food groups should we eat more of?

Which food group should make up the smallest part of our meals and diet?

When planning meals, it is important to make sure that they are balanced and suitable for the people who will eat them. For people who are preparing meals at home, providing balanced meals can be challenging for a number of reasons:

- People in a household may have particular likes and dislikes so it can be difficult to provide meals that everyone will eat.
- People are often short of time and cannot spend a long time planning meals.
- Many people eat foods out of the home and it is not always easy to know whether or not the ingredients they are made from provide a balanced meal (they may contain a lot of 'invisible' fat or salt).

ASSESSMENT FOR LEARNING

This could be a practical activity. For 1 and 2 below, make a timed plan (see page 9) and make some of the dishes you have chosen.

1 Using the Eatwell Plate, suggest a packed lunch that you or a friend could take to school. Remember to include foods from all the groups in the correct proportions.
2 Charleen is 14 years old and is overweight. Her mother has taken advice from a dietician and is helping her to eat more healthily with the aim of gradually losing some weight. Using the Eatwell Plate, suggest a breakfast, lunch and evening meal for Charleen.
3 Dietary guidelines suggest that a good way to make sure that a meal is balanced is to serve food that is a mixture of natural bright colours. Suggest three different meals that are a mixture of natural bright colours.

4 The food diary below shows the food eaten by a 28-year-old woman who works in an office as a secretary. She says that it is typical of what she eats most of the time.

Day 1	Day 2	Day 3	Day 4	Day 5
7am				
Doughnut Cup of coffee	Croissant Cup of coffee	A bowl of sugar-coated cornflakes and milk Cup of coffee	Croissant Cup of coffee	A bowl of sugar coated cornflakes and milk Cup of coffee
10am				
Two chocolate biscuits Cup of coffee	Two chocolate biscuits Cup of coffee	Three chocolate biscuits Cup of coffee	Two chocolate biscuits Cup of coffee	Slice of fruit cake Cup of coffee
12.30pm				
Two slices of pizza Bottle of cola	Bag of crisps Apple Bottle of cola	Egg and mayonnaise sandwich Bottle of cola	Ham sandwich Bottle of cola	Bag of crisps Satsuma Bottle of cola
4pm				
Two chocolate biscuits Cup of tea	Slice of chocolate cake Cup of tea	Chocolate éclair Cup of tea	Two chocolate biscuits Cup of tea	Two chocolate biscuits Cup of tea
6.30pm				
Takeaway chicken curry with rice Strawberry yogurt	Chicken pie with small salad Apple pie and cream	Spaghetti Bolognese, carrots and peas Ice cream	Fish and chips Yogurt	Steak, chips, peas and mushrooms Cheesecake with cream
10pm				
Cheese and biscuits Cup of coffee	Four chocolates Cup of coffee	Two chocolate biscuits Cup of coffee	Cheese and biscuits Cup of coffee	Three glasses of wine Two bags of crisps

a) Is this person's diet balanced? Give reasons for your answer.
b) Does the diet have too much or too little of any particular food groups? Give examples and reasons for your answer.
c) If this woman continues to have the same eating habits for a long time, what are the possible consequences for her long-term health?
d) What suggestions would you make to improve her diet? Give reasons for your answers.
e) Choose one of the days of the food diary, and say how you would change what was eaten. Give reasons for your answers.

ASSESSMENT FOR LEARNING

Using the Eatwell Plate, suggest two main meals that would be suitable for each of the following people.

1 Maria is 25 years old. She is an ovo-lacto vegetarian (she eats eggs and dairy products) and has just had her first baby. She is breast feeding the baby (see page 143).
2 Ryan is 18 years old and is training to run in a marathon in seven days time (see page 48).
3 Luke is 30 years old and has type 1 diabetes (see page 151). He has to have daily insulin injections.
4 Tom is 84 years old and is a widower. He likes to attend a senior citizens' lunch club. Suggest a meal that the club could plan for people like Tom (see page 138).

TOPIC 7

NUTRITIONAL NEEDS OF GROUPS

INTRODUCTION

Some people have a special dietary need, which means that they have to pay careful attention to what they eat. Dietitians are trained to give advice to people about special diets and help these people to manage their dietary needs well.

The topics that follow give information on different types of dietary needs, including their specific nutrient requirements and the types of foods that people can eat.

7.1 BABIES AND CHILDREN

DIETARY NEEDS

From the time we are born to the time when we become old, our need for different nutrients changes. When planning meals, in order to make sure that the right balance of nutrients is provided, we need to take into account the following things about the person we are providing food for:

- their age
- their size
- their state of health
- their stage of development
- their daily physical activities.

BABIES (BIRTH TO 12 MONTHS)

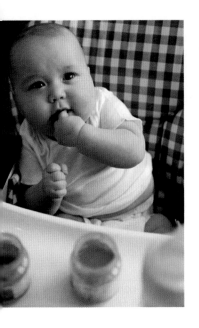

Newborn babies should only have milk for the first four to six months of their life.

Human breast milk is designed naturally to provide all the energy, nutrients and water that newborn babies need, except for the mineral iron. Newborn babies are born with a store of iron in their body (providing that their mother had enough iron in her diet when she was pregnant) which lasts about three or four months. Breast milk also enables babies to build up their immunity to disease and infections and is easy for the baby to digest.

If a baby cannot be breast-fed, then a specially made milk formula is given with a bottle.

After four to six months, small amounts of very soft foods are given to the baby as well as milk. This is called 'weaning'.

Different and larger amounts of raw and cooked foods must be introduced to the baby very gradually, so that it gets used to the textures, flavours and quantity of them and is able to digest them properly.

Foods that are known to cause allergies in some people, such as peanuts, wheat, egg, soya, shellfish, nuts and some fish, should be introduced very gradually into the diet, especially if someone in the family is known to have a food allergy. The general advice is to wait until the baby is at least 12 months old, and for shellfish, nuts and peanuts it should be much later.

The food should contain a good balanced variety of nutrients, including iron, so that the baby can continue to grow and get enough energy as it becomes more and more active.

Babies do not need to have added sugar or salt in their food or drinks. If they are given sweet foods and drinks they will continue to want them as they get older. This is not good for their long-term health, and the craving for sweet foods and drinks can be very difficult to stop.

YOUNG PRE-SCHOOL CHILDREN (ONE TO FOUR YEARS)

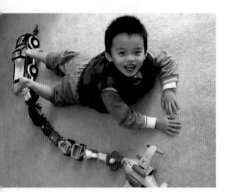

Pre-school children are rapidly growing and are usually very physically active as they are continually developing the skills of walking, running, climbing, playing and learning.

They need to have regular small meals and drinks to provide them with enough nutrients and energy throughout the day. At this age, they cannot easily eat large amounts of food in one go.

The dietary guidelines and Eatwell Plate (see page 67) do not apply in full to this age group as a diet low in fat and high in fibre would not give them enough energy.

It is particularly important that young children have enough nutrients.

Nutrient	Reasons why they are important to young children
Protein	They are growing rapidly at this age
Fat	To provide them with energy and fat soluble vitamins A, D, E and K. They should have whole cow's milk rather than semi-skimmed or skimmed as it provides more energy and nutrients. Fat is also needed for the development of the brain and nervous system
Carbohydrate	To provide energy, preferably from complex carbohydrate foods (which also supply other nutrients), such as potatoes, rice, pasta and bread, rather than sugar.
Calcium and vitamin D	For healthy bone and teeth development
Iron and vitamin C	To enable children to produce enough energy to keep up with their level of growth and activity
B vitamins	To enable children to produce enough energy to keep up with their level of growth and activity and help their nervous system and muscles to grow properly

At this age, eating habits become established, so it is important that parents and carers encourage children to do the following:

- try new foods to increase the range of foods they eat
- eat fresh and raw foods such as fruits and vegetables
- sit down at the table to eat so that they concentrate on and enjoy their meal
- drink water rather than sweetened drinks
- eat until they are full rather than being encouraged to eat everything on their plate – this will encourage them to recognise when their body tells them to stop eating, which will be very important for preventing over-eating and controlling their weight when they are older
- limit the number of sweets, crisps, biscuits and other snack foods that have limited nutritional value but lots of fat, sugar and salt.

At this age children can be gradually taught about where foods come from, how to prepare and cook them and how to enjoy them. This will build their knowledge of food and make it easier in the future for them to try new foods.

Children at this age can be fussy about what they eat and may refuse to eat certain foods. This can be very worrying for parents and carers who will naturally feel concerned about the child's health and development. Parents and carers need to encourage them to eat but try not to make this into a big issue as it will create more problems and the child may then refuse to eat as a way of asserting itself (trying to get its own way).

Parents and carers could try the following suggestions to tempt the child to eat:

- Encourage the child to help shop for, prepare and cook the food. This will make them feel involved in the whole process of eating.
- Serve very small portions so that the child does not feel overwhelmed by a large plateful of food.
- Give the child a small choice of foods so that they can decide what to eat.
- Serve the food in fun and interesting ways, such as some salad ingredients in the shape of a face.
- Invite a few friends to a meal to share the food.

SCHOOL-AGED CHILDREN (FIVE TO TWELVE YEARS)

This age group of children should be physically active and learning and developing skills. There is a danger that many children become physically inactive due to watching television, using a computer, staying indoors and sitting down and being driven to places in a car.

An increasing number of children in the UK are becoming overweight or obese because they eat a lot of energy dense foods, and do not take enough physical activity to use the energy that the food has supplied.

Their food should continue to provide them with a good variety and balance of nutrients, and they should have regular mealtimes and be discouraged from snacking and 'grazing' all day.

They need the nutrients listed in the charts on pages 88–90 for the same reasons. From the age of five years they can follow the dietary advice and Eatwell Plate guidelines, and do not need to have whole milk but can have semi-skimmed instead.

Children in this age group have 'growth spurts' (when they physically grow taller in a few weeks), and may be hungrier than usual when this happens. The food that they eat should provide them with plenty of protein as well as the minerals needed to make their bones grow. Physical exercise will help the bones take up minerals and become strong.

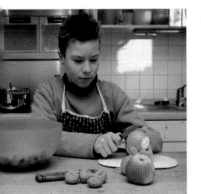

Children should continue to be encouraged to try new foods to develop their appreciation of foods. They should never be forced to eat something they do not like or made to eat everything on their plate if they say that they are full up.

As with younger children, this is an ideal age to provide them with knowledge about food and how to prepare and cook it. This will enable them to make more informed choices about what to eat when they are older.

ACTIVITY

1. Give two reasons why human breast milk is the most suitable for babies.
2. What does 'weaning' mean?
3. Why must babies have iron in their diet when they are weaned?
4. Why shouldn't babies and young children be given sugary foods and drinks?
5. Name three nutrients that are particularly important for young children.
6. Suggest three ways in which parents and carers can establish good eating habits in young children.
7. Why is it important that school age children have plenty of calcium in their diet and exercise?
8. Why is it a good idea to teach children about food and how to cook it?

7.2   TEENAGERS

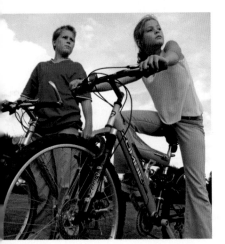

CHANGING FROM CHILD TO ADULT

At this stage of life, when the body is physically changing from that of a child to an adult, it is very important that the body receives a good, healthy balance of nutrients, following the Eatwell dietary guidelines (see page 67).

Growth spurts are usually sooner for girls and slightly later for boys. During this time they may be very hungry and need regular, well balanced and filling meals that provide them with energy. Teenagers can grow several centimetres in just a few months, so it is especially important that they have enough protein and calcium, vitamin D, iron, vitamin C, vitamin A and vitamin B to enable the bones, muscles and internal organs to grow properly.

Approximately between the ages of 15 and 20 years, teenage boys especially, develop muscle tissue in their arms, legs, chest and abdomen, and need a good supply of protein to enable this to take place.

Teenage girls especially need plenty of iron and vitamin C, to prevent them from becoming anaemic when they have their periods. The iron and vitamin C is also needed by both girls and boys to make sure that they are able to produce enough energy from their food and avoid feeling 'run down' and tired and becoming anaemic. This is particularly important as many teenagers have a tendency to sleep for less time than their body needs and they need to be able to concentrate when studying at school.

Teenage boys and girls need to make sure they have enough calcium, vitamin D and other minerals to enable their skeleton to develop normally and eventually reach peak bone mass. Milk provides a good source of calcium and other nutrients, but it is also available from green leafy vegetables, bread, cheese, yogurt, the bones of canned fish, nuts and seeds. Peak bone mass is when the bones have as much minerals in them as they can take and are at their strongest. Although it is not finally reached until about 30 years of age, most of the minerals are laid down in the bones during the teenage years, which is why teenagers should be encouraged to:

- eat a well balanced diet, including calcium and vitamin D-rich foods
- take regular load-bearing physical exercise such as walking, running, ball games, gymnastics and dancing as this stimulates the growing bones to take up minerals from the blood and lay them down in the bone tissue
- avoid drinking too many fizzy (carbonated) drinks (especially cola drinks) as research suggests that the phosphoric acid in these can prevent proper mineralisation of the bones.

Teenagers are often concerned about their looks and image, particularly their skin, hair and body size. Eating unprocessed, natural foods including fruit and vegetables, seeds and nuts and wholegrain cereals will provide a good range of vitamins and minerals that are needed to maintain the health of the skin, hair, nails and teeth.

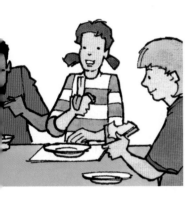

Limiting the intake of fatty, sugary and salty foods will help control body weight and size and will help to keep the heart and blood pressure healthy. Being physically active will help to maintain body size and prevent weight gain.

Teenagers need to eat regular, good quality meals. Breakfast is particularly important as it provides nutrients after the body has been resting, and it is known that most growth occurs when we are asleep, therefore by morning more nutrients are needed by the body to make up for what they have used during the night. Breakfast also helps teenagers to concentrate for longer when they are studying at school, especially if it contains foods such as wholegrain cereals or bread, fruit and porridge (which take longer for the body to process and so maintain the levels of glucose in the blood to provide energy) and protein foods such as milk and eggs.

ACTIVITY

1 Why is protein especially important for teenagers?
2 Why is it important that teenagers eat breakfast?
3 Why is iron especially important for teenage girls?
4 Name one good source of calcium for a teenager.
5 Name two good sources of calcium for a teenager who does not drink milk.
6 Explain why it is important for teenagers to eat a healthy, balanced diet.

ASSESSMENT FOR LEARNING

1 A secondary school has decided to employ a local catering company to prepare and cook school lunches for all its staff and pupils. The catering company wants to involve the pupils in the choice of foods for the menu, keeping within the dietary guidelines. As a group, suggest five different meals that you would want to be able to eat in the school dining hall. Give reasons for your choice and say how you have tried to keep within the dietary guidelines.
2 The data below shows the dietary reference values (see page 87) for three nutrients for teenage boys and girls.

Nutrient	DRV Boys 11–14 years	DRV Boys 15–18 years	DRV Girls 11–14 years	DRV Girls 15–18 years
Iron	11.3mg	11.3mg	14.8mg	14.8mg
Calcium	1,000mg	1,000mg	800mg	800mg
Protein	42.1g	55.2g	41.2g	45.0g

a) How much protein is needed by a 17-year-old girl?
b) How much protein is needed by a 17-year-old boy?
c) Why do you think there is a difference between the figures in a) and b)?
d) How much iron is needed by a 15-year-old boy?
e) How much iron is needed by a 15-year-old girl?
f) Why do you think there is a difference between the figures in d) and e)?
g) How much calcium is needed by an 18-year-old boy?
h) How much calcium is needed by an 18-year-old girl?
i) Why do you think there is a difference between the figures in g) and h)?

7.3   ADULTS AND SENIOR CITIZENS

ADULTS

Once people become adults, their body growth stops but they still need to eat a balanced diet to maintain the health of the body and to prevent the development of diet-related health conditions, such as heart disease and obesity.

Depending on the amount of physical activity that they take, adults need to try to maintain their body weight within a healthy range by balancing their energy intake with their activity levels. As people get older, the rate at which the body uses food for energy (metabolic rate) gradually slows down, and the amount of food that they eat will need to be adjusted accordingly. This is not easy to judge, and weight gain may occur gradually over a period of time.

Adults need to maintain the health of their skeleton by making sure that they have plenty of calcium and vitamin D in their diet and by taking physical exercise. Adult women also need to make sure that they have enough iron to cope with menstruation.

SENIOR CITIZENS (ELDERLY PEOPLE)

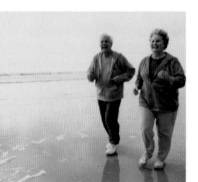

As the body ages, some of the systems in it start to slow down. The digestive system and the blood and circulatory system and some parts of the body start to wear out, such as joints between bones.

A healthy, balanced diet following the Eatwell guidelines (see page 67) will help to offset the effects of ageing. Sometimes doctors recommend that elderly people take vitamin and mineral supplements to help them.

Senior citizens who remain as physically active as possible and who continue to eat well balanced diets can enjoy their life and remain healthy.

The chart below explains which nutrients in particular are important for senior citizens.

Nutrient	Reasons why they are specially important
Calcium Vitamin D	• As the body ages, the bones naturally lose minerals and become weakened. This is known as osteoporosis (see page 79) and it can lead to the bones becoming very weak and brittle • Vitamin D is needed to absorb calcium in the body. Most vitamin D is made naturally in the body by exposing the skin to sunlight, but if an elderly person lives indoors most of the time (due to disability, immobility or being in a care home) they may not get enough vitamin D • It is recommended that people over the age of 65 years should take a vitamin D supplement • Calcium intake needs to be maintained to help slow down the effects of osteoporosis • This is especially important if an elderly person is unable to take much physical exercise to stimulate the bones to take up calcium

Nutrient	Reasons why they are specially important
Energy intake	• As the body gets older, it gradually has less lean muscle tissue and so the amount of energy needed each day goes down • Also, many elderly people tend to be less active so they do not need as much energy • It is important not to eat too many energy dense foods (fatty and sugary foods) because this may lead to obesity • It is recommended that elderly people stay as active as possible for as long as possible because this keeps the body weight down, helps them to sleep well and stimulates the appetite • However, if an elderly person has a very small appetite, they may need to have energy dense foods to make sure they have enough energy each day
Fibre and water	• The digestive system slows down as the body gets older, so it is important for elderly people to eat plenty of foods containing fibre, such as fruit, vegetables and wholegrain foods such as wholemeal bread, breakfast cereals, brown rice and pasta • This will help to prevent health conditions such as constipation and diverticular disease (see page 63) • Enough water should also be drunk every day to avoid dehydration and constipation and help the kidneys to work properly
Vitamin C and iron	• Anaemia can be a problem for many elderly people, because iron is not as well absorbed as the body gets older • It is important that they have enough iron-rich foods in their diet, such as red meat, liver, kidney, green vegetables, eggs, dried apricots, black treacle and molasses • They also need to have enough vitamin C to help absorb the iron from food and prevent the early signs of vitamin C deficiency – weakened blood vessels leading to small red spots of blood appearing under the skin
Antioxidants – vitamin C, E and A	• There is some evidence which suggests that having enough of these vitamins in the diet can help prevent age-related eye conditions in some elderly people
Sodium (salt)	• As the body gets older, the blood pressure often increases. It is important that the sodium/salt intake is carefully checked to avoid making this problem worse • Elderly people who live alone and have limited cooking facilities or abilities may rely heavily on ready-made meals from supermarkets. Some of these products have a high sodium/salt content, which can add to the problem of high blood pressure • If the sense of taste and smell has declined, elderly people may add more salt to their food to give it more flavour, which may raise their blood pressure. Alternative flavours such as herbs and spices should be used to avoid this
Vitamin B_{12}	• As the body gets older, it may not absorb vitamins such as B_{12} very well, and a deficiency of this vitamin is fairly common in the elderly • Research has suggested that a deficiency of vitamin B_{12} may be linked to gradual loss of memory in elderly people • Vitamin B_{12} is found in liver, shellfish, red meat, milk and fortified breakfast cereals • Some elderly people may need a supplement of vitamin B_{12}

For many senior citizens, undernutrition (where they do not receive enough of certain nutrients) may be a real problem, due to a variety of reasons.

Oral (mouth) problems

Senior citizens may have chewing and swallowing problems due to ill-fitting dentures (false teeth), loss of their own teeth, gum disease or the effects of a stroke or illnesses such as Parkinson's disease, which can cause swallowing difficulties.

Manual dexterity (being able to use the hands properly)

They may have arthritis in their hands (which causes the finger joints to swell, become very painful and twist out of shape) or frail skin which makes food preparation difficult. Or they may not be able to use their hands and arms because they have suffered a stroke or have Parkinson's disease.

Social problems

They may have lost interest in their food for a variety of reasons, such as loneliness and isolation, being widowed, living in a care home and losing their independence, ill health or being depressed.

They may not have the facilities or the ability to cook for themselves. This may especially be a problem for elderly widowed men who always had their meals prepared by their wife.

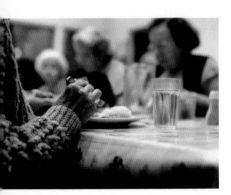

It may be difficult for them to go out and buy their food because they find walking and carrying heavy shopping difficult, they are disabled or good food shops may be some distance from where they live and transport to and from them may be a problem.

In many communities, voluntary groups and social services provide services to help elderly people to shop and eat well:

- Senior citizens lunch clubs where people can meet together in a social situation and eat a hot meal for a small price.
- Mobility buses collect elderly people and take them to shops, clubs or outings.
- 'Meals on wheels' where meals are delivered to elderly people's homes. These can either be frozen for later use or eaten on the day they are delivered.
- Food co-operatives buy fruits, vegetables and other foods and sell them from a van which travels to areas where senior citizens live.
- Home helps visit elderly people regularly in their homes and help them with shopping and cooking.

Poverty

Senior citizens may live on a very small income which means that they only have a limited amount to spend on food.

Poor absorption of nutrients

As the body gets older, changes in the digestive system take place, which may mean that some nutrients are not so well absorbed into the body. Certain medicines and drugs can also affect how well some nutrients are absorbed and can also affect how food tastes which can reduce the appetite.

Changes in the senses

When you eat, the sense of smell and taste work closely together to enable you to enjoy the food (think what food tastes like if you have a heavy cold and blocked nose). As the body gets older, we are less able to taste or smell food. This effect is worsened if the person has smoked for a number of years. This can reduce the appetite.

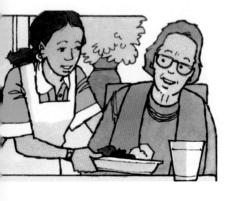

Help and advice

It is particularly important that senior citizens with health conditions such as diabetes and heart disease receive regular health checks and advice on their diet.

Very elderly people may need help with preparing their meals and with eating them and need to be cared for to make sure they also have enough to drink.

Often, elderly people have small appetites and may need to have small, but more regular meals.

ACTIVITY

1 Identify one nutrient that should be included in the diets of elderly people.
2 Explain why this nutrient is important.
3 What advice would you give to an elderly person who is no longer physically active but who wants to keep to a healthy weight?

ASSESSMENT FOR LEARNING

1 A local church is planning to set up a senior citizen's luncheon club to provide two-course hot meals for elderly people living in the area. The meals will be prepared and cooked in the church kitchen by volunteers and served to the elderly guests in the hall. Suggest three menus that the volunteers can make that will be enjoyed by the guests and will provide them with a good range of nutrients. Give reasons for your choices.

2 The table below shows energy and calorie needs for different age groups.

	KJ per day	Kcal per day
Age – males		
15–18 years	11,510	2,755
19–50 years	10,600	2,550
51–59 years	10,600	2,550
60–64 years	9,930	2,380
65–74 years	9,710	2,330
75+ years	8,770	2,100
Age – females		
15–18 years	8,830	2,110
19–50 years	8,100	1,940
51–59 years	8,000	1,904
60–64 years	7,990	1,902
65–74 years	7,960	1,895
75+ years	7,610	1,810

a) How many Kcals per day does a male aged 72 years old need?
b) How many Kcals per day does a female aged 70 years old need?
c) How many Kcals per day does a male aged 80 years old need?
d) How many Kcals per day does a female aged 77 years old need?
e) Which age group (males and females) in the chart above needs the most energy?
f) Explain why there is a difference in energy needs between adults and elderly people.

3 Plan a day's menu for an elderly person who wishes to have a healthy diet but who has a small appetite.

7.4 PREGNANT WOMEN

PREGNANCY AND DIET

During pregnancy women have to make sure that their diet supplies all the nutrients and energy required for the growing foetus (baby) and to maintain their own body. This does not mean that they need to eat twice the amount of food that they normally do! What it does mean is that they need to ensure that they have a balanced diet and that they have enough nutrients that are especially important at this time.

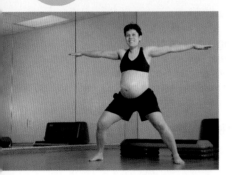

Calcium and vitamin D

During pregnancy the baby's skeleton gradually develops and the bones take shape, grow and become hardened with minerals. In the first few weeks the baby's skeleton is made of cartilage (a tough, flexible tissue) and, gradually, calcium starts to be laid down in the cartilage to turn it into bone. Most of the calcium is laid down in the baby's skeleton in the last three months of pregnancy.

The baby gets its calcium from the mother's blood supply. Therefore it is essential that the mother has enough calcium in her diet (see p. 90) to maintain her own bones as well as supply the baby. This is especially important for pregnant teenagers and young adults because their own skeletons are still developing and they will not yet have reached their peak bone mass (where the skeleton has a full supply of calcium and other minerals to make the bones strong).

Vitamin D is needed to absorb calcium in the body, so it is also essential that pregnant women have sufficient in their diet and are exposed to sunlight to enable their body to make vitamin D under the skin (see page 55).

If the mother does not have enough calcium or vitamin D during pregnancy, the baby will take calcium from her bones, which will then become weakened. This means that she may be at risk of developing osteomalacia (the adult form of vitamin D deficiency – see page 55) or osteoporosis when she is older (weakened bones due to a natural ageing process – see page 79).

Vitamin D is also found in liver, but pregnant women are advised not to eat liver, especially in the first few months of pregnancy because it contains high levels of vitamin A which could affect the baby's development.

Some pregnant women may require calcium and vitamin D supplements to make sure they receive enough. The doctor will advise if this is necessary.

Some foods and substances prevent calcium from being properly laid down in the bones, and should therefore be avoided during pregnancy. They include alcohol, caffeine (found in coffee, tea, cola, high energy caffeine stimulant drinks, chocolate and some pain relief tablets) and nicotine.

There is also evidence that the acids in carbonated (fizzy) soft drinks also prevent proper bone mineralisation.

Iron

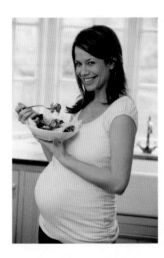

Iron is part of the haemoglobin in red blood cells. Haemoglobin picks up oxygen from the bloodstream and takes it to all the cells in the body to enable them to produce energy.

During pregnancy the volume of blood in the mother's body increases by 50 per cent. This is to enable her body to cope with the demands of the growing baby, by making sure she has enough energy and that the baby receives all the nutrients it needs to grow and develop properly.

In the last three months of pregnancy the baby needs to build up a store of iron in its body to last it for a few months after it is born while it has only milk and no other food. This is because milk contains very little iron, so it is vital that the mother has enough iron in her diet to make this happen.

The mother can make sure that she has enough iron by eating iron-rich foods (see page 58).

Vitamin C is needed to enable iron to be absorbed in the body, so the mother also needs to make sure that she eats foods rich in vitamin C (see page 53).

Folic acid (folate)

An intake of folic acid helps reduce the risk of the unborn baby developing defects in its spine such as spina bifida. This is a disabling condition where the spinal cord grows outside of the protection of the vertebrae (backbones). Women who plan to have a baby and pregnant women in the first three months of pregnancy are advised to take a folic acid supplement from the time they stop using contraception until the twelfth week of pregnancy.

Pregnant women are also advised to eat plenty of foods that contain folate (the natural form of folic acid) (see page 51).

Fibre

During pregnancy the woman's body produces hormones which make sure that the pregnancy develops normally. The hormones have a relaxing effect on the muscles of the intestines which means that they slow down and it takes longer for solid waste products from the digestion of food (faeces) to pass along the intestines and out of the body. This can cause constipation, especially in the later stages of pregnancy when the baby is becoming bigger.

Constipation can be very uncomfortable and it can be avoided by eating enough fibre (see page 63).

PREGNANCY AND WEIGHT

Often during the first three months of pregnancy women may feel sick and do not want to eat. This can be difficult to deal with and the best advice is to eat a little when they feel they can, eat as healthily as possible and drink plenty of water to prevent dehydration if they have been sick.

As the foetus gets bigger, it can cause pressure on the internal organs, such as the stomach. A pregnant woman may find she needs to eat frequent but small amounts of food to feel comfortable.

It is normal to gain some weight during pregnancy, some of which is fat that is stored so that the mother can use the energy from it to make breast milk and remain active after the baby is born. A careful check is made on weight gain during pregnancy to make sure the mother does not gain too much. The diet should contain only small amounts of energy dense foods such as fatty and sugary foods (snack foods, some ready-made meals, fried fast foods, pastries, cakes and biscuits, ice cream and sweets), as these will contribute to weight gain without providing many other useful nutrients.

FOODS TO AVOID DURING PREGNANCY

To protect the health of the mother and the development of the unborn baby, it is advisable to avoid certain foods during pregnancy, as the chart on the next page explains.

After the baby is born, and especially if the mother is breastfeeding, she needs to maintain a balanced diet in order to keep up with the demands of looking after a new baby. She especially needs to make sure that she has enough of the following:

- **calcium** – to provide enough to make milk for the baby to make its bones grow and to maintain the strength of her own skeleton
- **iron** – to replace any lost through bleeding during and after childbirth and give the mother enough energy to cope with the demands of breastfeeding and caring for a new baby
- **vitamin C** – to enable her to absorb iron

Food to avoid	Reason
Pâté – all types including liver and vegetable Soft cheeses – Brie Camembert and Chevre (goat's cheese)	These food products sometimes contain a type of bacteria called listeria which can cause illness in the mother and may harm the unborn baby
Soft blue cheeses	These may contain food poisoning bacteria which may cause illness to the mother and possible harm to the unborn baby
Raw or lightly cooked meat, especially food products made with raw minced meat	Meat and meat products should be cooked thoroughly all the way through to at least 70ºC in the middle
Liver, liver products and vitamin A supplements (cod liver oil)	Liver naturally contains a lot of vitamin A Supplements may give the body too much vitamin A Too much vitamin A may harm the unborn baby
Raw or partly cooked eggs or products that may contain them such as mayonnaise and mousse	These may contain a type of bacteria called salmonella, which can cause illness to the mother and possible harm to the unborn baby Eggs should be cooked until they are solid
Certain types of fish – shark, swordfish, tuna and marlin	These may contain high levels of the metal mercury which can affect the development of the unborn baby's brain and nervous system
Alcohol and caffeine	The baby may be underweight when it is born

ACTIVITY

1 Name two nutrients that women need when they are pregnant and explain why they are needed.
2 Suggest two good sources of each of these nutrients.
3 Why do pregnant women need to include fibre in their diet?
4 Suggest two good sources of fibre for a pregnant woman.

- **protein** – to enable the mother to make enough milk and help her body to recover from childbirth
- **energy** – breastfeeding requires energy to make the milk; some of this will come from the energy laid down as a fat store in the body during pregnancy and some will come from food
- **fluid** – women who breastfeed need to make sure that they drink plenty of water, especially during hot weather, so they do not become dehydrated.

Any weight gained in pregnancy will gradually be lost if a woman remains active and eats a balanced diet.

ASSESSMENT FOR LEARNING

1 The chart below shows the dietary reference values (DRVs) (see page 87) for protein, energy, vitamin C and calcium for an average, healthy woman aged between 15 and 50 years.

Nutrient	DRV	DRV when pregnant	DRV when lactating (breastfeeding)
Protein	45g	51g	56g
Energy	1,940kcals	2,140kcals	2,390kcals
Vitamin C	40mg	50mg	70mg
Calcium	700	700	1,250mg

a) What is the DRV for protein for a pregnant woman?
b) What is the DRV for vitamin C for a lactating woman?
c) How much extra calcium does a lactating woman need compared to a pregnant woman?
d) Why is the DRV for calcium different for a lactating woman compared to a pregnant and non-pregnant woman?
e) Why is the DRV for protein different for a pregnant woman compared to a non-pregnant woman?
f) Why is the DRV for protein different for a lactating woman compared to a pregnant woman?
g) Why is the DRV for vitamin C different for a lactating woman compared to a pregnant woman?
h) Why is the DRV for energy different for a lactating woman compared to a pregnant woman?

2 Plan a healthy, high fibre breakfast and evening meal for a pregnant woman. Explain why the menu you have chosen is particularly suitable for a pregnant woman.

7.5 PEOPLE TRYING TO LOSE WEIGHT

LOSING WEIGHT AND EFFECTS ON HEALTH

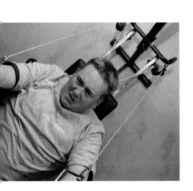

Being overweight or obese can make people more likely to develop health conditions such as:

- heart disease
- diabetes
- high blood pressure
- osteoarthritis (painful and damaged joints) especially in the hips and knees.

It can also have other health consequences such as:

- feeling low or depressed about how they look
- problems having surgery because of the fat under the skin
- breathing difficulties because of the weight of the body fat on the chest
- skin rashes and infections because of bacteria becoming trapped under folds of fat.

If a person is overweight or obese, losing weight has great benefits for how they feel about themselves, how they look and for their short and long-term health, as it reduces the risk of developing the health conditions listed above.

Many people who want to lose weight are often tempted to try a commercially advertised weight loss diet plan or product which suggests that they can lose weight quickly. But many people are disappointed to find that the weight loss can take quite a long time, or that when they stop the diet they put weight back on very quickly and sometimes end up heavier than they were before.

The important thing to remember about body weight is that it takes quite a long time to put on weight and therefore it will take quite a long time to lose weight permanently. This means that someone must be very determined and motivated to lose weight and may need the support of family, friends or a weight loss club.

The only way to lose weight successfully is to use up more energy in physical activity every day than you take in from food. If you can increase your activity levels by taking exercise, the process of losing weight will be quicker, but you must eat a balanced diet to maintain the health of the body.

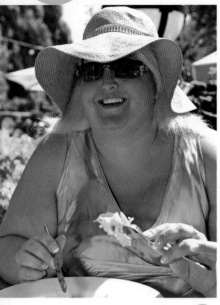

Often, people gradually put on weight because over a period of time they have changed their eating habits and lifestyle, without realising that they have increased their energy intake and reduced their energy output. This can happen because:

- They may eat more fast foods out of the home (which tend to be fried or have a high fat or sugar content).
- They may eat more snack foods in between meals.
- They may have gradually increased the portion sizes of their food.
- They may have a less active job.
- They may spend more time in a car or watching the television.

CHANGING EATING HABITS

People who have decided that they need to try to lose weight need to change their eating habits and lifestyle by following the suggestions below:

- Eat fewer energy dense foods such as sweet and fatty foods (potato crisps, chocolate bars, biscuits, cakes, pastries, fried foods, chips, pizzas, ice cream, cream, sweet fizzy drinks and mayonnaise). These foods contain a lot of fat and/or sugar and therefore provide a lot of energy. If the energy is not used doing physical exercise, the person will put on weight.
- Eat more low energy foods such as fruit, vegetables, salads and wholegrain cereals and cereal products such as wholemeal bread, brown rice and wholegrain pasta. Fruits and vegetables have a high water content and low energy value and are filling. Wholegrain cereals and cereal products have a high fibre content which can make you feel full.
- Change their methods of cooking by grilling, steaming and baking food instead of frying it. This reduces the fat content and energy value of the food.
- Use low fat versions of products such as cheese, milk, spreads and sauces to reduce the energy value of the diet.
- Use low sugar versions of products such as fizzy drinks and yogurts to reduce the energy value of the diet.
- Be more active by walking, riding a bicycle, going swimming, climbing the stairs, running or playing a sport in order to increase energy output and use up energy that is stored as fat in the body.

Once the weight has been lost, it is important to maintain healthy eating habits and physical activity in order to maintain the new weight.

ACTIVITY

1 Identify two benefits of losing weight.
2 Describe three things a person can do to try and lose weight.
3 Explain why grilling, steaming and baking foods are better cooking methods to use when someone is trying to lose weight.

7.6 VEGETARIANS

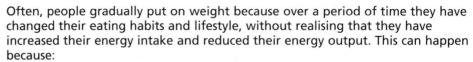

WHAT IS A VEGETARIAN DIET?

Vegetarians are people who choose not to eat meat, poultry, meat and poultry products (sausages, cooked meats, gelatine), offal such as liver, kidney and heart or fish and seafood, where an animal, bird or fish has had to be killed. They base their diet mostly on plant foods.

There are various reasons why people follow a vegetarian diet, including:

- They do not want to eat the flesh of a dead animal, bird or fish.
- They disagree with raising and killing animals, birds and fish for food because they think it is either cruel or a waste of land, water, energy and food which could be used to feed more people instead.
- They consider a vegetarian diet to be healthier than a meat-eating diet.
- They have religious reasons not to eat meat, poultry or fish.

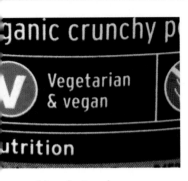

Manufacturer's own
labelling of vegetarian food

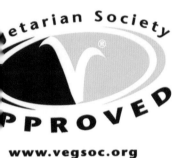

www.vegsoc.org

The Vegetarian Society
Approved logo, part of an
independent accreditation
scheme for vegetarian food

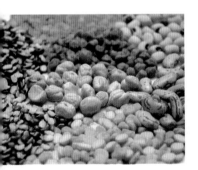

Lentils are a vegetarian
source of iron

Food labelling

Vegetarians can usually identify whether or not a food is suitable for them to eat, as food manufacturers often use words such as 'meat free', 'suitable for vegetarians/vegans' and 'free from dairy foods/eggs'. Or they may use a symbol to indicate this, like the ones shown here.

TYPES OF VEGETARIANS

There are three main types of vegetarians:

1 **Lacto-ovo vegetarians**: They will eat the products from animals or birds, where the animal or bird has not been killed or physically suffered in any way. Lacto means that they will eat dairy foods, such as milk and milk products (cheese, butter, cream and yogurt). Ovo means that they will eat eggs.
2 **Lacto-vegetarians**: They do not eat eggs but will eat dairy foods.
3 **Vegans** (sometimes called strict vegetarians): They do not eat any animal food products at all, even if the animal has not been killed to provide the food product. Vegans eat only plant foods such as cereals, nuts and seeds, pulses (peas, beans and lentils), as well as fruits and vegetables.

NUTRITIONAL NEEDS OF VEGETARIANS

Vegetarians should make sure that they eat a variety of foods every day in order to provide them with a balance of nutrients. It is especially important to make sure that they have a sufficient supply of certain nutrients, including:

Iron

Iron that is found in meat and meat products is most easily absorbed by the body, but as vegetarians do not have this source of iron in their diet, they must rely on the iron found in plant foods. The iron in plant foods is less easily absorbed because some of it becomes firmly attached to other natural substances in plant foods which prevent it from being absorbed.

Vitamin C

Vitamin C helps the body to absorb iron, so it is important for vegetarians to make sure that they include plenty of fresh fruit and vegetables in their diet to provide this.

The plant and non-meat sources of iron include:

- wholegrain cereals and cereal products such as brown rice, wholemeal flour, pasta and bread, breakfast cereals with iron added to them (fortified)
- green vegetables such as spinach, kale, cabbage, watercress, spring greens, okra, broccoli, brussels sprouts and peas
- dried fruits such as apricots and figs
- lentils and beans such as soya beans
- nuts such as pistachios, almonds, hazelnuts and cashews
- seeds such as sunflower, pumpkin and linseeds
- egg yolk
- cocoa and dark, plain chocolate
- black treacle and molasses.

Vegetarians with particularly high iron requirements, such as someone recovering from an accident or operation, a teenage girl or woman with heavy periods, a woman who is pregnant or just had a baby or an elderly person, may be advised by their doctor to take an iron supplement so they do not become deficient and develop anaemia (see page 58). It is possible to buy vegetarian iron supplements, such as blackstrap molasses capsules.

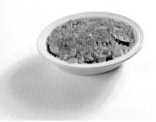

Grilled vegetable bake

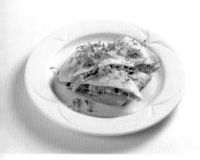

Bean quesadillas

Protein

Foods that contain high biological value (HBV) protein (see page 39) and provide all the essential amino acids that the body needs are mostly found in animal foods. For a lacto-ovo vegetarian, there should be no problem in getting enough HBV protein if they regularly eat eggs and milk products.

Plant foods, except for soya beans and quinoa (this is how you say it: keen-wah) contain low biological value (LBV) protein (see page 39). This means that they are missing one or more of the essential amino acids. This is not a problem if a mixture (combination) of plant proteins is eaten every day, e.g:

- lentil soup with bread
- nut roast containing a variety of nuts, seeds and cereals such as bread
- nut stir fry served with egg-free pasta
- vegetable and soya bean curry served with brown rice and naan bread
- nut butter spread on toasted bread
- hummus with pitta bread.

This is particularly important for vegans (strict vegetarians), especially vegan children, as plant foods can be quite filling and enough need to be eaten to provide them with sufficient protein.

It is also possible to buy soya milk, tofu and tempeh (both made from soya beans) which provide a good source of protein and minerals, and soya products such as desserts, custards, yogurts and textured vegetable protein (TVP) which can vary the diet.

Quorn is a man-made vegetarian food product which is made from a mycoprotein. This is a type of fungus (like mushrooms) which is grown under special conditions and turned into a variety of products such as burgers, minced quorn, quorn pieces, sausages and ready meals. It contains a good source of protein, but it is not suitable for a vegan diet because during manufacture egg white protein is used and some quorn products contain milk protein. It has a low fat content and contains some fibre.

B vitamins

Most of the B vitamins can be obtained from a variety of foods (see page 49).

However, Vitamin B_{12} is mainly only found in animal foods, so for a lacto-ovo vegetarian, dairy products and eggs are a good source. For vegans the sources of food are limited to fortified foods such as yeast extract, soya milks, sunflower margarine and breakfast cereals. Vegans can also take vitamin B_{12} supplements.

VEGETARIAN DIETS AND DIETARY GUIDELINES

A well planned vegetarian diet can be a very healthy diet and will meet the advice of the dietary guidelines, especially if it contains a high proportion of fresh fruits and vegetables (at least five-a-day) and cereals and cereal products. Vegetarian diets are often low in saturated fats and high in fibre.

Vegetarian food can also be very interesting, tasty, colourful and varied by making use of the wide variety of fruits and vegetables, beans, nuts and cereals that are available.

ACTIVITY

1 What is a lacto vegetarian?
2 What is a lacto-ovo vegetarian?
3 What is a vegan?
4 Suggest two nutrients that may be lacking in a vegetarian diet and identify a range of foods that can supply these nutrients.

ASSESSMENT FOR LEARNING

1 Plan a breakfast, lunch and evening meal for a lacto-ovo vegetarian. Include some good sources of iron and vitamin C in the meals. Give reasons for your choices.

2 You have invited three people (two friends plus a guest of one of them) to come for a meal and have planned the following menu: prawn salad starter, lamb lasagne with roasted vegetables and strawberry mousse (set with gelatine).

You find out the day before that the guest who is coming with your friend is an ovo-lacto vegetarian, and so cannot have any meat, meat products, poultry or fish. You do not want the guest to feel awkward, so you decide to adapt the menu so that she can enjoy the meal.

Explain how you would adapt the menu and give your reasons.

7.7 COELIACS

COELIAC DISEASE

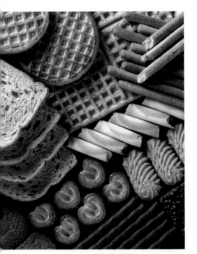

A coeliac (this is how you say it: see-lee-ack) is a person whose body cannot tolerate the protein gluten, which is found in wheat, barley, oats and rye and any food product made from or containing these (biscuits, bread, crackers).

If they eat these foods, the gluten damages the lining of their small intestines, which prevents other nutrients from being absorbed into the body. This condition is called coeliac disease.

The symptoms of coeliac disease include:

- Weight loss – the person is not absorbing food properly, so cannot get enough energy which means that their body has to use up its fat stores for energy.
- Lack of energy and tiredness – not enough food is absorbed to provide energy.
- Diarrhoea – the damage to the intestines means that the faeces (solid waste products from the digestion of food) are not properly made.
- Anaemia – not enough iron or vitamin C is absorbed.
- Poor growth in children – the body cannot absorb enough protein and other nutrients to make it grow.
- General malnutrition – not enough nutrients are absorbed, especially calcium, folic acid, vitamin D and iron.

Food that coeliacs cannot eat

Coeliac disease is permanent. It cannot be cured, but the damage to the intestines and the malnutrition can be improved if no foods containing gluten are eaten. It can occur at any age, but it is usually diagnosed either when a baby is weaned (starts to eat solid food) or later in life as an adult.

Food labelling

Coeliacs can usually identify whether or not a food is suitable for them to eat, as food manufacturers often use words such as 'gluten free', or they may use a symbol (called the cross-grain) to indicate this, as shown here.

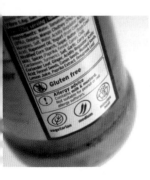

The chart on page 115 shows which cereal foods contain gluten. If you are a coeliac, it is very important to check the ingredients labels of foods carefully as often they contain small amounts of cereal products that may contain gluten.

There is a charity organisation in the UK called Coeliac UK (**www.coeliac.org.uk**) which supports coeliacs by providing them with information about the disease. It publishes a list of foods and drinks that contain gluten and those that are gluten free to help coeliacs choose a healthy diet.

The chart on the next page shows which plant foods coeliacs can eat.

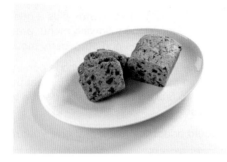

Cake made with polenta

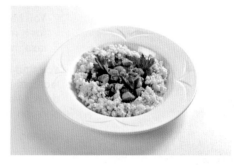

Spicy chicken with quinoa

Name of food	What it is used for
Agar	An alternative to gelatine to set cold desserts
Almonds	Used in bakery products such as biscuits and cakes as an alternative to flour
Amaranth	A plant that is used as an alternative to wheat and other cereals
Buckwheat	To make flour and noodles
Carageenan	Used as a thickener and stabiliser in foods
Cassava/manioc/ tapioca	Used as a cereal and a thickener
Chestnuts	Ground up and used as a flour
Corn (maize)	Used as a flour and thickener
Linseeds (flax)	Can be added to foods such as breakfast cereals to increase nutritional intake and energy
Gram flour	Made from chickpeas and used in a variety of dishes as an alternative to wheat flour
Millet	Often used as a muesli and added to other foods
Mustard	Used as a seed, an oil or a flour in a variety of dishes
Polenta	Made from boiled corn (maize) meal and used in cakes, puddings and savoury dishes
Potato flour	Can be used in cakes, pastries and biscuits and as a thickener
Peas, beans and lentils	Made into flours for a variety of dishes
Quinoa	Used in baking and as an alternative to rice or couscous
Rice	Many types – used either whole, flaked or ground in many dishes
Sago	Used as a thickener or pudding
Sorghum	Used as a cereal or a source of syrup
Soya flour	Used in biscuit, cake and pastry making
Urd/urid	A flour made from lentils

There are several food products specially produced for coeliacs:

- Group 1: Naturally gluten-free foods such as those listed in the chart above. Most of these do not stretch to allow doughs to rise very much when baking, which means they are alright for cakes, biscuits and some pastries, but not so good for bread.
- Group 2: Foods made to be gluten free by removing almost all the gluten from wheat flour. This produces wheat starch which has a good flavour, but does not produce a stretchy dough, so the bread made from it tends to have a close texture. Some coeliacs cannot tolerate these products because they still contain a small amount of gluten.

Coeliacs need to make sure that they avoid foods that contain gluten and that they choose a variety of fresh foods, including fruits and vegetables, meat, poultry and fish, dairy foods and eggs.

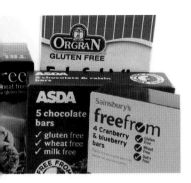

Specially produced gluten-free food products

ACTIVITY

1 What is a coeliac?
2 Why can coeliacs not eat gluten?
3 Name two symptoms of coeliac disease.
4 Identify (list) three foods that coeliacs should avoid eating.
5 Identify three gluten-free plant foods that coeliacs can eat.

ASSESSMENT FOR LEARNING

Imagine you have invited three people (two friends plus a guest of one of them) to come for a meal and have planned the following menu: tomato soup with bread rolls, chicken pie with carrots, mashed potatoes and broccoli, and apple sponge pudding with custard.

A few days before, you find out that the guest who is coming with your friend is a coeliac, and so cannot have any food with wheat in it. You do not want the guest to feel awkward, so you decide to adapt the menu so that he can enjoy the meal.

Explain how you would adapt the menu to remove any wheat from it and use an alternative and give your reasons.

7.8 DIABETICS

WHAT IS DIABETES?

Diabetes (see also page 77) is a health condition where the amount of glucose in the blood is too high. In a non-diabetic person, the amount of glucose in the blood is kept at normal levels by a hormone called insulin. Insulin acts a bit like a key and 'unlocks' the cells to let glucose in. In a diabetic person either they do not produce any insulin or their body is unable to use it.

A low level of glucose in the blood is called hypoglycaemia (hypo = too little, glyc = glucose, aemia = blood), while a high level is called hyperglycaemia (hyper = too much). This means that the body's cells cannot get their energy from glucose (because it is 'locked out' and cannot get into the cells) and the glucose stays in the blood, which over a period of time causes damage to the blood vessels, especially in the following parts of the body:

- The eyes – the tiny blood vessels at the back of the eye become affected and this eventually leads to blindness.
- The hands and feet – these start to feel 'tingly' then become numb because the blood is not reaching them properly. A serious infection can set in, which may result in a foot or leg having to be amputated (removed by surgery).
- The internal organs such as the kidneys.

Diabetics are also more likely to develop heart disease, strokes (blood clot in the brain) and high blood pressure.

There is no cure for diabetes, but it can be managed by medication and diet.

There are two types of diabetes.

Type 1 diabetes

This is also called insulin dependent diabetes. It usually develops in childhood or early adulthood. In this type of diabetes, the body's immune system (which protects the body from infection and diseases) appears to turn against itself, and in doing so, it destroys the special cells in the pancreas (a small organ situated just behind the stomach) that produce insulin. Without the insulin, the body quickly develops symptoms including the following:

- Weight loss – the body cannot use the glucose from food to get energy so it has to use up its fat stores.
- Thirst – the extra glucose in the blood makes the person feel very thirsty.
- Increased need to go to the toilet to pass urine – due to drinking more.
- Tiredness – due to being unable to use the glucose for energy.
- Blurred vision – due to the effects of extra glucose in the blood vessels in the eyes.
- Itching of the genitals – due to the glucose which goes into the urine as the body tries to get rid of it.

Type 1 diabetes is treated by:

- giving the patient regular insulin injections
- eating a healthy balanced diet.

Patients are taught how to inject themselves which they may have to do several times a day. They also learn how to check their blood sugar levels by a simple blood test (from a drop of blood collected from the finger) and urine tests (using a special stick which is dipped into the urine and shows how much glucose is there).

Injections are timed according to:

- the amount and type of food eaten
- how much and what type of exercise is taken.

The aim is to keep the blood glucose levels as stable as possible.

Type 2 diabetes

This is also called non-insulin dependent diabetes. Type 2 diabetes develops either because the body does not produce enough insulin or the insulin does not work properly.

This type of diabetes used to be only seen in elderly people, but in the last few years there has been a large increase in the numbers of much younger people developing the disease in the UK and many other countries. It is thought that there are approximately 0.4 million people in the UK with Type 1 diabetes and 1 million with Type 2. It is thought that 120 million people in the world have Type 2 diabetes, and it is predicted that this number will double by 2010.

There are also many more people with symptoms of diabetes who have not yet been diagnosed. These numbers are increasing each year and are thought to be linked to more people being overweight and obese due to eating too many sugary and fatty foods, not enough fibre and not exercising enough.

Type 2 diabetes is treated (and the development of it prevented) by:

- eating a healthy, balanced diet (following the Eatwell Plate guidelines)
- increasing physical activity and exercise
- losing weight
- tablets or injections to control the blood sugar levels – for some patients.

MANAGING THE CONDITION AND STAYING HEALTHY

The advice given to diabetics is the same that is recommended for the whole population: eat a balanced diet that is based on starchy complex carbohydrate foods, plenty of fresh fruit and vegetables and is low in salt, fat and sugar.

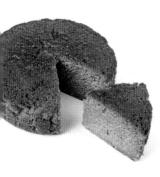

Carrot cake is naturally sweet

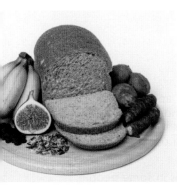

Foods a diabetic should choose

In order to do this, diabetics should follow the advice below:

- A small amount of sugary foods can be eaten, preferably as part of a meal. There is no need to buy specially made diabetic food products such as cakes and biscuits as these can be expensive and often contain a lot of fat.
- Many cake and biscuit recipes can have their sugar content reduced without greatly affecting the finished results. This is a good way of reducing sugar intake. Also, naturally sweet foods, such as grated carrot, could be added to cakes and biscuits instead of some of the sugar.
- Some fruit products, such as dried fruits and concentrated fruit juices, contain quite high levels of sugar, so should be limited in the diet. Fruit juice drinks usually have added sugar, so it is better to choose non-concentrated fruit juice.
- It is possible to buy canned fruit, such as peaches, in fruit juice instead of syrup.
- Honey contains a lot of sugars, so its use should be limited.
- Complex starchy foods, such as potatoes, yams, cassava, rice, bread and breakfast cereals (non-sugary ones), which are broken down slowly in the body should be eaten to provide energy.
- Wholemeal/wholegrain complex carbohydrate foods (wholemeal bread, porridge oats, brown rice and pasta) are broken down to glucose slowly in the body (unlike sugary and non-wholemeal foods, which put glucose into the bloodstream very quickly). This means that the body has time to deal with the glucose going into the blood, which makes managing the diabetes much easier with less damage to the body.
- Diabetics are at greater risk of developing heart disease so they need to control their intake of fat and salt and increase their intake of vegetables and fruits to provide them with antioxidants (see page 55) such as vitamins A, C and E which help prevent heart disease.
- They should choose to eat lean meat and poultry, fish, beans and pulses instead of fatty meat or hidden fat in meat products such as pies, fried foods and pasties.
- They should choose low fat dairy products and limit the amount of oil and fat used in cooking.
- They should choose low salt foods and limit the amount of salt added to foods and naturally salty foods such as bacon, ham, cheese, yeast extract and salted fish. This will help the kidneys to work well and help prevent high blood pressure.
- Diabetics need to get into the habit of reading food labels to make sure that they know what food products contain, and seek advice from their doctor or dietitian if they are unsure. Many foods contain 'hidden' sugars which are sometimes listed under their chemical names – sucrose, dextrose, fructose, maltodextrin, glucose syrup – so they need to be able to recognise these.

ACTIVITY

1 Name the two types of diabetes.
2 Describe the changes that a diabetic person needs to make to their diet in order to manage their condition.
3 Explain why a person with diabetes should eat more wholemeal and wholegrain foods such as bread, rice and breakfast cereals.

ASSESSMENT FOR LEARNING

1 Suggest what a diabetic person could choose to eat instead of the foods listed in order to help control their diet.

- White bread
- White rice
- Frosted cornflake breakfast cereal
- Concentrated orange juice drink
- Sultanas and raisins
- Canned peaches in syrup
- Fried egg, sausage and chips

2 Plan an evening meal that is suitable for a diabetic. Include a good source of wholegrain complex carbohydrate in or with the meal. Give reasons for your choices.

7.9 FOOD ALLERGIES AND INTOLERANCES

WHAT IS A FOOD ALLERGY?

A food allergy is the body having an allergic (bad) reaction to a food or an ingredient in a food. An allergen is the substance in the food which causes the reaction. It makes the body produce a substance called histamine (a natural chemical of the body) and other chemicals that cause the abnormal reaction. You may have heard of people taking anti-histamine tablets to control the symptoms of hay fever, which is a similar type of allergy to pollen from grasses and flowers. The histamine gives the body a range of symptoms.

An allergic reaction to food can happen within a few seconds, minutes or hours after eating or touching a food. It can cause the person to have symptoms such as:

- skin rashes
- itchy skin and eyes
- runny nose
- swollen lips, eye lids and face
- wheezing and coughing.

For some people, an allergic reaction can be very sudden and very serious. It can lead to a condition known as anaphylactic shock (this is how you say it: anna – fiy – lak – tick), where the person will develop swelling in their throat and mouth, find it difficult to swallow or speak and may then collapse and could die if they are not treated very quickly by a doctor.

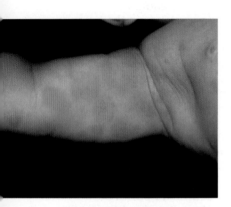
This child has had an allergic reaction to a food

The following foods are known to cause allergic reactions in some people:

- eggs
- peanuts and other nuts
- seeds
- strawberries, kiwi fruit and other fruits
- seafood – prawns and shrimps.

WHAT IS FOOD INTOLERANCE?

Some people develop food intolerances (sometimes called food sensitivity), which give them a variety of symptoms such as:

- pain and bloating in the abdomen
- diarrhoea
- nausea (feeling sick)
- muscle and joint aches and pains
- general tiredness and weakness.

Food intolerance is much harder to diagnose than food allergy. The usual way to diagnose it is for the person to stop eating the food which is thought to be a problem and see if they start to feel better. If they do, the food is tried again and if symptoms come back it is clear that the person cannot tolerate it.

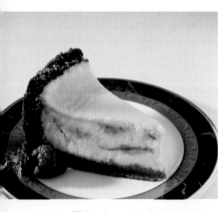
This cheesecake contains lactose

An example of food intolerance is lactose intolerance where a person cannot digest the milk sugar lactose. This gets broken down by bacteria in the large intestine instead which causes abdominal pain, diarrhoea, flatulence (wind) and nausea (feeling sick). A person with this condition needs to avoid all foods that contain milk, milk products and lactose, or buy lactose-reduced and lactose-free products.

Some people cannot tolerate chocolate or cheese because these foods give them a migraine (very bad headache). Other people cannot tolerate certain food additives because they give them asthma, nausea or they are unable to concentrate and become hyperactive.

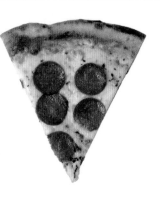

This pizza contains wheat and lactose

Some people are intolerant to wheat because of its gluten content, but they may not have full coeliac disease (see page 149). They may find that when they eat wheat they feel bloated, tired, have diarrhoea and nausea and that these symptoms go away when they either reduce the amount of wheat they eat or stop eating it all together. Wheat is used in many processed foods and food products, so it is quite challenging to remove it from the diet.

MANAGING FOOD ALLERGIES AND INTOLERANCE

Once someone knows which foods they are allergic or intolerant to, they can make sure they avoid them. Providing they eat a balanced diet, they should remain healthy and without symptoms.

People who are likely to have an anaphylactic shock should always carry an epipen which they can inject into their arm or leg if they feel a reaction happening. The epipen injects adrenaline into the body which acts quickly to stop blood vessels leaking, relaxes muscles in the lungs to make breathing easier, helps the heart beat and helps stop swelling in the face and lips. The person must be taken to hospital very quickly for medical treatment.

People with these conditions need to make sure that they do the following:

- Read food labels very carefully to check for ingredients they may be allergic or intolerant to. Most food labels will show whether or not they contain certain ingredients that are well known to cause allergies or intolerances. The names of allergens are often 'hidden', e.g. another word for peanuts is 'ground nuts' and this may be used in a ready meal as ground nut oil. Medicines also sometimes use ingredients that may cause an allergic reaction. For example, 'arachis' is the Latin name for peanuts and might be found in some tablets.
- Ask in a restaurant what is in the food if they eat out. This is very important because often foods that may cause an allergic reaction are prepared in the same place or with the same equipment as other foods and this may be enough to cause a reaction in very allergic people.
- Let friends, teachers, employers and work colleagues know about their condition in case they are taken ill and show them where the epipen is kept and how to inject it.
- Contact food manufacturers and supermarkets and ask for a list of products that contain foods that can cause allergies. Most companies can provide this information.

ACTIVITY

1 What is a food allergy?
2 Name two foods that are known to cause allergies in some people.
3 What is food intolerance?
4 Name two foods that are known to cause intolerance in some people.
5 List two things a person who knows they have a food allergy should do to avoid problems.

ACTIVITY

You and two friends are going out for the day and are taking a packed lunch.

One of your friends is intolerant to wheat.

Plan four food items that would be suitable for the packed lunch that you could all eat.

7.10 CORONARY HEART DISEASE

WHAT IS CORONARY HEART DISEASE (CHD)?

CHD is a disease in which the coronary arteries, which give the heart muscle its oxygen, become blocked (see also page 74).

In the figure of the heart here you can see the coronary arteries covering the heart muscle (they look like tree branches).

- At **A** you can see a healthy artery cut across – it is clear so that blood can flow through it easily.
- At **B** the artery is partly blocked so the blood cannot flow through very easily – this would cause pain when the person tried to run or walk fast. The pain would disappear when the person rests. This type of pain is called angina.
- At **C** the artery is almost completely blocked and the blood would not be able to pass through and deliver oxygen to the heart muscle. This would cause a heart attack where some of the muscle is permanently damaged (as shown by the red area).

During a heart attack, a patient would have the following symptoms:

- a severe crushing pain in the centre of the chest which spreads to the arms, throat, jaw, back and abdomen – the pain will not go away with resting
- breathlessness
- weakness
- feeling sick
- feeling sweaty.

If only a small area of muscle is affected in a heart attack, it is likely that the person will survive. If a lot of muscle is affected, the person may die.

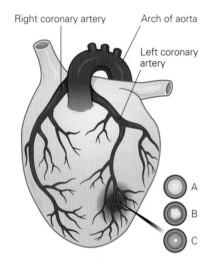

Right coronary artery   Arch of aorta

Left coronary artery

A
B
C

Source: based on
www.healthyheart.nhs.uk

What causes blockages in the arteries?

The walls of the artery become narrow and blocked with a build up of fatty substances (called atheroma). Then the blood starts to become semi-solid because some of the small cells (platelets) stick to each other and the wall of the artery – this is called a thrombosis.

The blocking of the coronary arteries is a gradual process that may take several years. There are a number of risk factors (see also page 75) which make this more likely to happen, which are set out below.

The amount of cholesterol in the blood

Cholesterol is a fatty substance which is made in the liver from the fats we eat in our food. It is needed for several jobs in the body. Cholesterol is carried round the body attached to special proteins called lipoproteins.

If we eat a lot of saturated fats from foods such as meat, cheese, butter, suet and solid vegetable fats, we make more cholesterol than the body needs and it gets carried around the body by lipoproteins called LDLs (low density lipoproteins) and is deposited in the artery walls. Some people call this 'bad' cholesterol.

If we eat more unsaturated fats from foods such as vegetable, nut and seed oils (sunflower, rapeseed and olive oil), less cholesterol is made and it is carried round the body by lipoproteins called HDLs (high density lipoproteins). It does not get deposited in the artery walls and some people call this 'good' cholesterol.

It is possible to have the cholesterol levels in the blood measured to find out how many LDLs and HDLs we have. Some people naturally have high levels of LDLs and they may need to take special medicine to prevent this causing heart disease.

Other factors

- Smoking cigarettes causes the blood to become 'sticky' so it is more likely to form a blockage.
- High blood pressure puts a strain on the arteries and the heart. It may be partly due to eating too much salt.
- Being overweight or obese puts a strain on the heart and blood vessels.
- The heart is a muscle and it needs to be exercised to make sure that it works well. Exercising also puts more oxygen into the bloodstream which makes the heart work more efficiently.
- Fruit and vegetables contain substances (antioxidants) and fibre which help prevent damage to the artery walls by keeping blood cholesterol levels low and preventing other chemicals in the blood (pollutants from the air or water) from doing damage. These foods are also low in fat.
- Fibre from foods such as oats, wholemeal bread, pasta and brown rice helps to lower LDLs and therefore reduce cholesterol levels in the blood.

HOW MANY PEOPLE HAVE CHD?

CHD is the most common cause of death in the UK. It kills over 100,000 people a year and approximately 2.5 million people have the condition. The numbers of deaths from CHD have actually fallen since the 1970s, which may be due to fewer people smoking and better medical care (more people recovering from heart attacks). However, many more people are overweight and obese now and are at a high risk of developing CHD, so it is possible that these figures could increase. Also, more and more young people are developing the condition.

There are many ways to lower the risk of developing CHD:

- Eat a balanced diet following the Eatwell Plate dietary guidelines.
- Eat more fruits and vegetables and fibre.
- Choose low fat foods such as skimmed or semi-skimmed milk and milk products, lean meat and white fish.
- Grill or bake foods rather than fry them to reduce the fat content.
- Trim the fat off foods such as meat and poultry.
- Reduce the amount of fat spread on foods such as bread and toast.
- Stop smoking.
- Take more physical exercise to strengthen the heart and keep weight down.
- Try to lose weight if necessary.
- Reduce salt intake by using alternative flavours such as herbs and spices and cutting down on snack foods, ready meals and shop bought cakes and biscuits which contain baking powder which is a source of sodium (see page 59).

ACTIVITY

1 What do the letters CHD stand for?
2 What are the symptoms of CHD?
3 What happens to the heart muscle when the body has a heart attack?
4 What is cholesterol?
5 Why is it better to eat more unsaturated fats than saturated fats?
6 Why is it important to eat more fruits and vegetables?
7 Identify two risk factors for developing CHD.
8 Describe the changes that a person with CHD should make to their diet.

ASSESSMENT FOR LEARNING

1 The local health centre is putting up a display on CHD. Plan and prepare some posters giving advice on healthy eating for people with CHD or how to avoid developing CHD.

Include recipe and meal suggestions. Give reasons for your choices.

2 Imagine you are preparing a two-course evening meal for four people. Two of the people have CHD and have been told to reduce their fat intake to help lower their blood cholesterol levels. One of them also has high blood pressure.

Plan a menu showing how you have taken into account the dietary needs of the two people with CHD.

3 The graph below shows death rates from CHD in different countries in 2001.
   a) Which country had the highest death rate from CHD?
   b) Which country had the lowest death rate from CHD?
   c) Suggest why some countries have a much higher death rate than others.
   d) Which gender (male or female) has the highest death rate from CHD?

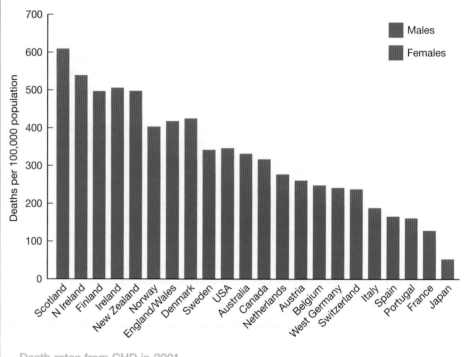

Death rates from CHD in 2001

Source: www.skyaid.org

TOPIC 8

FOOD CHOICE

Have you ever thought about why you choose to eat the foods that you do?

Many people take food for granted because there is plenty available to choose from and they do not stop to think very much about why they choose some foods and not others.

In fact, there are many reasons that influence why we choose the food we eat, and the chart below illustrates some of these.

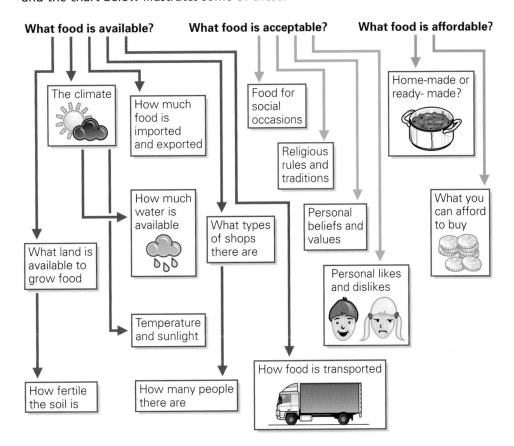

| 8.1 | SOCIAL AND ECONOMIC DIVERSITY |

ECONOMIC DIVERSITY

One of the most important influences on what people choose to eat is what they can afford to buy. Economic diversity means the differences between the amounts of money that different groups of people have to live on. In the UK there are some very rich people and some very poor people, and in between, there are many people who have just enough to live on.

Very poor people will find it difficult to pay for all the basic things they need to live: a home, heating and lighting, clothing, transport and food. Certain things, such as rent, electricity and gas bills must be paid, otherwise they will be taken away, so people have to find the money to pay for them. They may have to cut down on the amount they spend on food, which may mean buying cheaper food products which often contain a lot of fat, sugar and salt, rather than healthier foods which are often more expensive.

Rich people are able to pay for all their basic needs, including food, and have money left over for luxuries, including eating out.

People who have just enough to live on for all their basic needs, including food, may have to reduce the amount they spend on food when the prices of other items, such as their rent or mortgage, electricity, gas and petrol go up.

Here are some suggestions for producing meals on a limited budget:

- Use cheaper cuts of meat, such as shin of beef and neck of lamb.
- Use alternative and cheaper protein sources to meat or add them to make the meat go further, such as beans and pulses.
- Make your own food rather than buying ready-made meals.
- Use produce that is in season, such as fruits and vegetables, and preserve some of it if you can (freezing).
- Take advantage of special offers in the shops – money off, 'buy-one-get-one-free', three for two.
- Use supermarket own brands and some of their 'value lines'.
- Collect and use money-off vouchers from newspapers, magazines and leaflets delivered to your home.

SOCIAL DIVERSITY

Social diversity means the differences between people's opinions, which leisure activities they enjoy, who they socialise (are friends) with, and how important certain things (sport, clothes, friends, jobs, religion, music) are to them.

Food plays an important part in social diversity and is often used as:

- a gift (a box of chocolates or bottle of wine)
- a way of socialising (going out for a meal at a restaurant, having a takeaway with friends, sharing a cup of tea or coffee)
- a reward (a child given a sweet for good behaviour)
- a way of demonstrating your status (buying expensive bottles of wine or cuts of meat or prestigious foods such as caviar and smoked salmon).

ACTIVITY

1 Identify (list) some of the ways in which supermarkets try to help people on low incomes to buy their food.
2 Carry out a price survey on a range of food products (from the most expensive to the cheapest), such as ready-made shepherd's pies, vegetable soups, chicken curries. Compare the different products according to price, quantity and quality of ingredients, type and amount of packaging and style of labelling. Which do you think is the best value and why?
3 Read the case study below and carry out the activities following it.

Four students aged 19 years are moving into a house together and have a limited amount of money to spend on food each week. They like to cook their own food rather than buy it ready-made and want to eat together for most of their evening meals to save costs. They live near a street market that sells fresh fruit, vegetables, fish and cheese.

Plan a week's evening meals for the students that will be low cost, interesting, filling and nutritious. Give reasons for your choices and explain how they can save money when buying the ingredients and on fuel when cooking the meals.

8.2 CULTURAL AND RELIGIOUS DIVERSITY

Our food choices are influenced by many things. Some of the most important are the culture, religion, traditions and celebrations that we are brought up with. As well as keeping us alive, food is an important part of our social needs and is an essential part of many religions, celebrations and festivals.

CULTURE

The word 'culture' is used to describe:

- our way of life
- our patterns of behaviour as individuals, members of groups and society
- what makes us different from other people
- what we know and believe
- our laws and morals
- our customs and habits
- what we have inherited from our ancestors.

The term 'food culture' is a very important part of the general culture of a community and is used to describe the following.

HOW people choose to eat	WHAT people choose to eat	WHY people choose to eat	WHEN people choose to eat	WHERE people choose to eat
Using their hands?	Which foods they like	For an everyday meal?	At regular mealtimes?	At home?
Using knives, forks, spoons, chopsticks, sticks, plates, leaves?	Which foods they do not like	For a special occasion?	How often?	At a restaurant?
Sitting at a table?	Which foods they know are safe to eat	As a snack?	In between meals?	In front of the TV?
Sitting on the floor?	Which foods they know	To prepare themselves for a sporting event?	Only when they are hungry?	In bed?
While walking?	Which foods they do not know and have never tried	For a medical reason?	Whenever they want to?	At work?
Alone or with others?	How much they eat	As a treat or a comfort food?		In their car?
				Outdoors?

Every generation of people make changes to their culture, so gradually over time, certain aspects of the culture are altered. Traditions are usually preserved, but how they are actually carried out may be changed.

Culture is learned from the time we are born and we are often not aware of how much it influences what we do. It is just part of our normal behaviour (going to school, driving on the left, celebrating a birthday, talking about the weather, eating certain foods and not others).

Culture has values. Some behaviour is seen as being good (obeying the law, helping others less fortunate than you, not being anti-social to your neighbours) and some is seen as being bad (stealing, lying, hurting someone, cheating).

ACTIVITY

1 Identify (list) three activities that food culture includes.
2 What does socialisation mean?

Socialisation is the name given to the process of passing on culturally valued behaviours from one generation to the next.

Food culture is also learned from birth and includes:
- which foods are acceptable to eat and which are not
- which foods are considered good and bad for you – often the bad foods are highly desirable!
- what is an acceptable way to eat our food and what is not.

In the UK food culture has seen lots of changes in the last 50 to 60 years, as the chart below shows.

What has changed	What people used to do	How it has changed	Effects of these changes
Where our food comes from	Many people used to grow some of their own food	Most people buy their food from shops	Many people do not know how food is grown or where it comes from
How we buy our food	Buy their food fresh every day from markets and individual shops as many people did not have refrigerators or freezers	Most people buy all their food together once a week from supermarkets and store it at home in refrigerators and freezers	Many small shops and markets have gone out of business because they cannot compete with supermarkets Many foods have additives put in them to make them last longer
How we prepare our food	Most people cooked their meals from fresh ingredients at home Most women stayed at home to look after their families and were responsible for buying and cooking the food	Many meals and ingredients are sold ready-made and only need to be heated up Many women work out of the home and have a limited amount of time to shop for, prepare and cook food	Many people do not know how to cook or know what is in the food they buy ready-made More convenience and ready-made foods are available to save people time and effort All family members may be involved in food preparation
What we eat	Many people ate fairly simple, traditional meals, mostly at home Choices of foods were fairly limited to what could be grown in each season and what could be imported from other countries Foods were sold with very little packaging	Many snack foods are eaten between meals Many ready-made meals are bought Many people eat fast food which they buy outside the home People have tried foods from other countries when they have travelled abroad Many more foods are available and many are imported A lot of food packaging is used, much of which is plastic	Many people eat too much fat, sugar, salt and protein and not enough fruit, vegetables and fibre Many people expect food to be highly flavoured and coloured Foods from other cultures have become very popular and a normal part of UK culture A lot of foods are imported and eaten out of season Importing and packaging food causes damage to the environment and uses up lots of non-renewable energy

What has changed	What people used to do	How it has changed	Effects of these changes
Where we eat	Most people ate food at home, often at the table with other people	Many people eat out in restaurants, cafes and fast food shops Many people eat their food out of the home in the street, in their cars, in front of the TV and often alone	Eating out has become a normal part of UK culture The catering industry has grown very large with lots of different types of places to eat Many people do not regularly eat together at home as a family
When we eat	Most people ate regular meals throughout the day Food shops had set opening hours and did not open late or on Sundays	Food can be bought at any time of the day and night People in a household often have different working hours and eat at different times of the day or night	People may over-eat because food is available all the time and from many places Eating lots of snack foods throughout the day may lead to weight gain

ACTIVITY

1 Identify (list) one thing that has changed in the last 50 years about:
   - the way we buy our food
   - the way we prepare our food
   - what we eat
   - where we eat
   - when we eat.
2 Identify (list) one effect of each of the changes that you have identified above.

RELIGION

Food is an important part of religion and spiritual ritual for many different faiths. Most religions have a set of dietary rules or laws. These rules are often linked to traditional celebrations or times of the year.

The chart overleaf lists some of the main religions and their dietary rules.

Religious faith	Dietary rules
Buddhism	Most Buddhists are vegetarian and believe that any violence or pain given to others will be reflected on to you
	Some Buddhists avoid meat and dairy products
	Fasting is practised by Buddhist monks in the afternoon
	Buddhist monks and nuns cannot grow, store or cook food and must rely on food given to them by believers
Christianity (including Roman Catholic, Orthodox and Protestant)	Fasting (going without food for a period of time) is sometimes observed and is believed to improve spiritual discipline and to act as a reminder about people who regularly face starvation or malnutrition
	Before Easter many Christians observe Lent, where they give up certain foods for 40 days and nights. On Good Friday some may avoid eating meat
	Christmas is celebrated as a feast day with traditional foods such as turkey and mince pies
Hinduism	Hindus do not eat meat from certain animals, such as beef or pork, and avoid foods that may cause pain to animals when they are made
	A Hindu saying is 'food is God (Brahman)', and they believe that food contains certain energies that are absorbed by people when they eat the food
	Hindus try to avoid violence or pain to any living thing and so vegetarianism is encouraged but is not compulsory
	Certain foods, such as duck, are prohibited in some countries but not others
	Certain foods, such as onions, garlic and alcohol, are thought to excite the body and may affect a Hindu's search for spiritual enlightenment, and so these foods are either avoided or only eaten occasionally
	Dairy foods are considered to enhance spiritual purity
	In some communities fasting is practised
Islam	Muslims have a set of dietary laws which are found in the Qur'an, the holy book of Islam. The rules set out what is halal (lawful) in a Muslim's life, including food, particularly meat and poultry
	To make meat and poultry halal, an animal or bird has to be slaughtered in a ritual way known as 'Zibah', which requires that:
	• the animal or bird has to be alive and healthy at the time of slaughter
	• the animal or bird has to be killed by a Muslim with one single, clean cut to the throat, while a special dedication (called tasmiya or shahada) is recited
	• all the blood must be drained from the carcase (dead animal or bird)
	Unlawful foods are called 'haram', and include pork, pork products such as gelatine, alcohol, foods that contain emulsifiers made from animal fats, frozen vegetables with sauce, some types of margarine, drinks that contain caffeine and breads that contain dried yeast
	Ramadan is the ninth month of the Islamic calendar and during this time Muslims are required to fast during daylight hours. The fasting helps to teach Muslims self-discipline and generosity and to remind them of the poor
	Usually one meal (known as suhoor) is eaten just before sunrise and another (known as iftar) is eaten just after sunset. Different Muslim families and friends often come together to eat during this time
	At the end of the month, a big celebration, known as 'Eid-ul-Fitr' takes place for the breaking of the fast. Gifts are given and parties are held. A set amount of money must also be given to charity to help poor people buy new clothes and food

Religious faith	Dietary rules
Judaism	Food is a very important part of the Jewish religion. 'Kashrut' is the name given to Jewish food laws which were written more than 2,000 years ago
	'Kosher' means that a food is allowed to be eaten because it is 'clean'. Only fish with scales and fins and animals that chew the cud and have cloven (split) hooves, such as cows and sheep, may be eaten
	Anything 'unclean' (such as pork and shellfish) is strictly forbidden and called 'trefah'
	Foods must be prepared in the right way in order to be kosher – animals must be slaughtered correctly
	Dairy foods and meat must not be prepared or eaten together, which means that there must be separate preparation areas and cooking equipment for these foods
	On Saturdays Jewish law forbids any work, so the main meal is a slowly cooked stew, known as cholent. It is prepared the day before and left on a low heat
	Fasting is part of Judaism. On Yom Kippur, the Day of Atonement, Jews fast from dusk till dusk
	Jewish feast days include Rosh Hashanah and Passover, which remembers the birth of the Jewish nation. Bitter herbs are eaten to remind Jews of the suffering of the Israelites under Egyptian rule
Rastafarianism	Rastafarians eat strictly according to 'I-tal' which means that food must be natural and clean. They do not eat pork and only eat fish that is no longer than 30cms long.
	Rastafarians eat plenty of vegetables and fruits and use coconut oil to cook food. They do not drink alcohol, milk or coffee but do drink herbal teas
Sikhism	Many Sikhs are vegetarian
	On special days certain foods are eaten at the temple
	By eating together, Sikhs show that they are all equal
	Some Sikhs do not drink alcohol, tea or coffee

 ## TRADITIONS AND CELEBRATIONS

Throughout the world, food plays a main part in any celebration, no matter what culture or religion people belong to. Food is used to make friends by eating and talking together and helps to reinforce the bonds between people in a community.

Celebrations can include:

- the birth of a child and birthdays
- coming of age
- engagements to be married
- weddings and wedding anniversaries
- retirement from work
- remembering the life of a person who has died
- the end of a war or time of crisis in a country or community
- the building of an important facility in a community – a well to supply fresh water, a factory to provide jobs, a shopping centre, a community centre
- a special achievement – in sports, education, for bravery
- a special event in the year – the New Year, midsummer, Christmas.

TOPIC

9

HOW AND WHY FOOD IS COOKED

DIFFERENT WAYS TO COOK FOOD

Many foods are cooked before they are eaten, and there are several different ways to cook food.

ACTIVITY

The chart below gives the reasons why food is cooked. Match the pictures of food to the right reason.

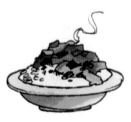

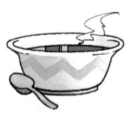

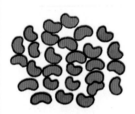

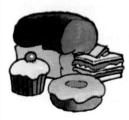

Reason for cooking food	Example of food
1 To destroy harmful bacteria in foods	Think of some foods that could give you food poisoning if they were not cooked properly
2 To develop the flavour of foods	Think of some foods that have a really good flavour once they have been cooked
3 To make food easier to bite, chew, swallow and digest	Think of some foods which are much easier to eat when they have been cooked
4 To make foods more appealing and attractive to eat	Think of some foods which you would not want to eat raw, but would if they were cooked
5 To give people a variety of foods by using different cooking methods	Think of one food and different ways in which you can cook it
6 To give people hot food when the weather is cold	Think of some foods that you would find comforting to eat when the weather is very cold
7 To destroy natural poisons in some foods and so make them safe to eat	Clue: this food is red, it comes from a plant and is an ingredient in chilli con carne
8 To enable foods to rise, be thickened, dissolved and set when preparing a recipe	Think of some recipes where you must have heat to make them work and get the right result

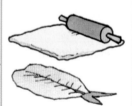

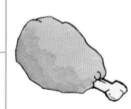

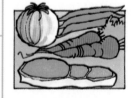

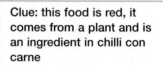

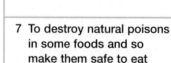

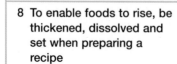

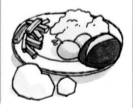

9.1 THE TRANSFER OF HEAT TO FOODS

WHAT IS HEAT?

Heat is a type of energy. All materials (solids, liquids and gases), including foods, are made up of very small particles called atoms. Atoms join together to form molecules. When these molecules receive energy, they start to vibrate and move quickly. This causes heat to be produced and the faster the molecules move the more heat is produced.

The heat is passed from one material to another by three different methods called conduction, convection and radiation:

- Conduction is the passing of heat through solid materials such as metals and food.
- Convection is the passing of heat through a gas or a liquid.
- Radiation is the passing of heat through space without the use of a solid, liquid or gas.

Conduction and convection

Here is a diagram of a pan of potatoes in water on a gas hob.

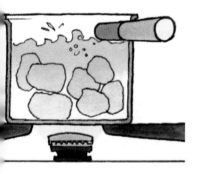

Energy from the burning gas is transferred to the metal of the pan.

The energy from the burning gas causes the molecules in the metal one by one to vibrate and knock against each other and as they do so, heat is produced. This is called conduction of heat.

The heat energy from the metal passes into the cold water and the water molecules start to move around very quickly in circular movements called convection currents. You can see this happening when you heat up a pan of water. As they do so, more heat is produced. In thicker liquids, such as sauces, the convection currents are much slower, so the mixture must be stirred to speed them up and stop the sauce cooking and sticking at the bottom of the pan and becoming lumpy. (Convection currents also happen in an oven as the air is heated up and rises then falls as it cools down.)

The heat from the water passes into the potatoes, and the potato molecules start to vibrate and move and heat is produced by conduction. The heat in the potatoes cooks the starch inside them and the potatoes become soft.

Some materials conduct heat through very easily and quickly. We say they are good conductors of heat. Metals and water are examples of good heat conductors. This is why baking sheets and pans are made of metal because the heat passes quickly into the food and cooks it quickly and effectively. It is also why you should be very careful not to allow your skin to come in contact with very hot water or steam, as they can cause serious burns.

Some materials do not conduct heat very well. We say they are poor conductors of heat but they are good insulators because they prevent heat from coming through. Wood, plastic, cloth (wool and cotton), still air and glass are insulators. This is why wooden spoons, plastic pan handles and oven gloves made of thick cotton cloth are used to protect your hands from being burned when you are cooking. Oven doors often have a double layer of glass with still air in between to enable you to see what is happening in the oven without burning yourself.

ACTIVITY

1 Name a method of cooking that uses conduction to transfer heat to food.
2 Name two materials that are good insulators.
3 Why might you choose to use a wooden spoon when you are stirring a hot mixture in a pan on the hob?
4 Explain what would happen if you did the following:
  a) removed a hot baking tray from the oven using a wet dishcloth
  b) removed a hot baking tray from the oven using a dry tea towel
5 Why would a cake baked in a glass dish take longer to cook than one baked in a metal cake tin?
6 Why is it important to always stir a sauce as it is cooking in a pan?

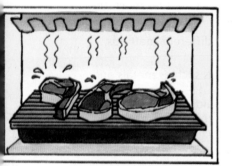

Radiation

Here is a diagram of lamb chops being grilled.

The heat energy from the grill is passed to the lamb chop by radiation. Radiation is the transfer of energy through space, which happens because of invisible electromagnetic waves. There are different types of these, including infrared rays and microwaves.

Infrared heat rays are absorbed by an object they reach (in this case, a lamb chop) and create heat inside the food, which cooks it.

ACTIVITY

The diagrams below show foods being cooked. Match them to the correct answer to identify and describe how heat is transferred to the food.

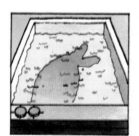
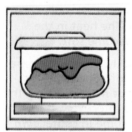
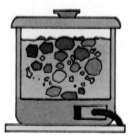

How is the heat transferred?

The electric heating element transfers heat to the slow cooker by conduction. The heat is transferred to the food by conduction and then by convection.

Heat transfers from the hob to the pan by conduction then to the contents of the pan by convection.

Heat is transferred from the electric heating element to the oil by conduction, then by convection to the food.

Heat passes to the surface of the food by radiation. The inside of the food then heats up by conduction.

The heat is transferred from the gas flames to the oven by convection. The heat is transferred from the metal baking tray to the food by conduction.

The microwaves cause the food molecules to vibrate and give off heat and the heat then passes through the food and to the dish by conduction.

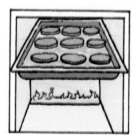
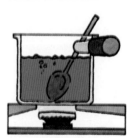
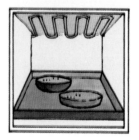

RESEARCH ACTIVITY

Sometimes glass, china or plastic dishes in which food is cooked in a microwave oven become hot. Microwaves do not cause this (because they pass through these materials), so how have the dishes become hot?

Cooking food in a microwave oven is another example of heating food by radiation. Microwaves are given off by a magnetron inside a microwave oven. The microwaves are absorbed by the food and make the food molecules vibrate very fast so that they give off heat which cooks the food.

Microwaves pass through materials such as glass, paper, china and plastics. The microwaves do not heat up these materials.

Microwaves are reflected back to the magnetron from metals. This will damage it and so metals should never be used in a microwave oven.

ASSESSMENT FOR LEARNING

Look at the statements below and on a piece of paper, put a tick ✓ against all the ones you can do. If you can tick them all, well done! Make sure you can remember them in case you are asked to repeat them.

I can...

- ☐ Name one method of heat transfer
- ☐ Describe what convection is
- ☐ Give an example of when radiation is used to cook food
- ☐ Give an example of a cooking method that uses conduction
- ☐ Give an example of a cooking method that uses convection
- ☐ Explain why it is a good idea to use a wooden spoon when stirring a hot mixture in a pan on the hob
- ☐ Describe how heat is transferred to a tray of biscuits in the oven
- ☐ Describe how heat is transferred to a pan of potatoes on the hob
- ☐ Name two materials that are good conductors of heat
- ☐ Identify three materials that are good insulators of heat
- ☐ Identify the parts of a microwave oven and explain what they are for

9.2 GRILLING, FRYING, ROASTING, BAKING AND BARBECUING

GRILLING

Grilling is a fast method of cooking. It transfers heat to food by radiation (see page 168). It causes fat in foods such as meat to melt and drain away. This reduces the fat content of the food, so grilling is a healthier cooking method than frying.

Food that is to be grilled should be up to 3.5cm thick. If it is any thicker, the heat will take too long to reach the centre of the food and the outside will be overcooked.

Meat that is to be grilled should be tender, such as rump beef steak, lamb chops or pork chops, as grilling will not tenderise tougher cuts of meat.

Poultry should be cut into pieces such as legs, drumsticks and breast fillets to make it easier to fit under the grill and allow the heat to cook it thoroughly.

Grilling can be carried out in a gas or electric cooker, with a special infrared electric grill or a combination microwave oven with a grill.

Frying

Frying involves cooking food in hot fat or oil. Food can either be deep fried in a large pan or electric deep fat fryer with oil that is several centimetres deep or shallow fried in a frying or sauté pan with a little fat or oil.

Heat is transferred to the food both by conduction (see page 167) from the pan and convection (see page 167) from the hot oil.

Foods that are fried soak up some of the fat or oil. This increases their fat content and energy value. After cooking, they should be drained carefully and allowed to stand on absorbent kitchen paper for a few minutes after frying to remove excess oil.

For both types of frying, the following rules should be followed:

- Some foods such as fish, meat, fruit and vegetables should be coated in a batter (made from egg, milk and flour) or egg and breadcrumbs. These form a protective layer over the food as it fries to protect it from the high temperatures used in frying and prevent it from overcooking. When the food is put into the hot oil, the egg protein coagulates (becomes solid), and with the other ingredients in the coating forms a crisp outer layer.
- Make sure the oil is hot enough before adding the food, so that it starts to cook straightaway. If it is not hot enough, the food will soak up the oil and become greasy and heavy. Most foods are deep fried at about 180°C. Electric fryers have a thermostat to control the temperature. A cooking thermometer should be used to check the temperature of a pan of oil.
- Never drop the food into hot oil.
- Do not allow the oil to become too hot or it will smoke and rapidly catch fire.
- Do not put too much food into the hot oil at the same time, otherwise the oil will cool down too much and the food will soak it up and become soggy and greasy.
- If a pan of oil catches fire, turn off the heat and cover the pan with a lid or very thick damp cloth to exclude oxygen. Never add water to burning oil and do not try to carry it out of the kitchen until it has cooled down.

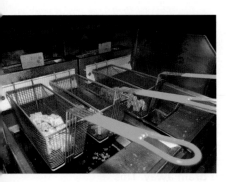

Deep frying

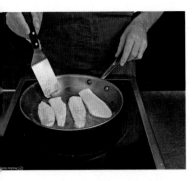

Shallow frying in a frying pan

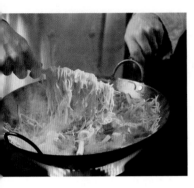

Stir frying

- Oils that are used for frying should be strained and filtered after being used to remove bits of food that have dropped into the oil. This will keep the oil in good condition.
- Oil should only be re-used a few times because every time it is heated up, some of the oil molecules break up and start to affect the flavour, shelf-life and ability of the oil to be heated to high temperatures. It is also bad for your long-term health to eat foods cooked in old oil as the broken up oil molecules may lead to the development of heart disease and some cancers.

Some foods, such as minced meats, can be dry fried. This means heating them gently in a frying pan without oil until the fat they contain starts to melt and cooks the food. This can be done when making a Bolognese meat sauce.

Stir-frying is a type of frying that is traditionally carried out using a wok. It is used as a method of cooking in countries such as China, Japan and Thailand. It is important to make sure that the wok is hot before you start cooking. A very little oil is put in and used to quickly cook the finely chopped ingredients such as fish, vegetables and meat. If the food in the wok becomes dry during frying, you can add a little water instead of more oil to carry on the cooking. This will prevent the food from burning and sticking to the wok, and will avoid the need to add more oil.

Stir-frying is a quick method of cooking and, as it uses only a little oil and the food does not have to be heated for very long (which means that vitamins are not so easily lost), it is a healthy method also.

ACTIVITY

1 What is the difference between deep frying and shallow frying?
2 Why do some foods need to be coated in batter or egg and breadcrumbs?
3 Why must the oil be hot enough before adding the food?
4 Why must you not allow the oil to become too hot?
5 What should you do if a pan of oil catches fire?
6 Why should you only use oil for frying a few times before throwing it away?
7 Why is stir-frying a healthier method of cooking than deep or shallow frying?
8 How is heat transferred to foods when frying?

ACTIVITY

Make a list of foods or recipes made from the following food groups that are suitable for shallow, deep, dry or stir frying.

- Meat (only tender cuts such as steaks and chops)
- Poultry
- Fish and fish products
- Dairy foods (e.g. foods made with cheese or eggs or batter)
- Cereal products (e.g. battered products, bread and bun products)
- Fruits and vegetables (e.g. fritters)

ROASTING

Roasting involves cooking foods in a hot oven with a little oil, and occasionally turning the food as it cooks to allow it to become crisp on all sides.

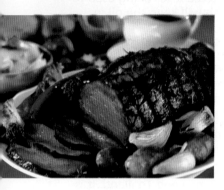

Roasted food

The heat is transferred from meat by conduction (see page 167) from the roasting pan and also from any bones that are in the meat or metal skewers that are placed into the meat.

Roasting causes water to evaporate from the food, which concentrates the flavours in the food. This makes foods such as roasted vegetables to have a good, robust flavour and colour.

As high temperatures are used, meat which is to be roasted should be tender. Tough cuts of meat will not tenderise by this method of cooking.

When roasting a meat or poultry joint, it is important to make sure that it is cooked right through. A guide to how long you should roast meat and poultry for is shown below. You should weigh the joint first then follow the cooking times.

Type of meat or poultry	Length of cooking time (when meat is put into a hot oven)
Poultry	For every ½ kg: 20 minutes + an extra 20 minutes
Lamb	For every ½ kg: 20 minutes + an extra 20 minutes
Pork	For every ½ kg: 35 minutes + an extra 30 minutes
Beef	For every ½ kg: 20 minutes + an extra 20 minutes
A joint that contains stuffing	Add an extra 10 minutes for every ½ kg, whatever the meat or poultry

It is important to choose the right type of meat joint for roasting so that the cooked meat is tender. The chart below shows the names of suitable roasting joints of meat.

Type of meat	Names of roasting joints
Poultry (chicken, turkey, duck, pheasant)	Whole bird, leg quarter, breast, turkey breast crown, poussin (very small chicken), drumstick, thigh
Lamb	Leg, shoulder, breast, best end of neck (crown roast), loin, neck fillet, chops
Pork	Leg, fillet, spare ribs, chops, belly, hand, shoulder
Bacon	Gammon, collar
Beef	Silverside, topside, sirloin, fore rib, ribs

Spit roasting means cooking food over an open fire or flames, while turning the food slowly so that it is evenly cooked. This method was used over many hundreds of years to cook meat and fish and is still used for some special events. Modern rotisseries are used to cook chickens, for example. These are usually electric and the chickens are placed on large metal skewers, which transfer the heat to the food by conduction, and rotated in the heat to ensure even cooking.

ACTIVITY

1 Why do roasted foods have a good flavour?
2 Why must meat be tender to be roasted?
3 Why must you cook meat or poultry for the correct length of time when roasting?
4 How is heat transferred to food when roasting?

ACTIVITY

Make a list of foods or recipes made from the following food groups that are suitable for roasting.

- Meat and poultry
- Fruits and vegetables

BAKING

Baking is cooking foods in a hot oven without fat or oil. The heat of the oven causes foods such as cakes, bread, Yorkshire puddings, choux pastry and scones to rise and then set. It is important to make sure that the oven is hot before putting these foods in to cook, so that the process of rising starts straightaway. For example, when making Yorkshire puddings, the water in the milk that is added to the batter mixture turns to steam in the oven and pushes up the mixture causing it to rise. The oven must be hot enough to create enough steam quickly for this to happen or the Yorkshire puddings will be flat and heavy.

In gas ovens, the top of the oven is usually the hottest and the bottom of the oven the coolest, so it is important to make sure that foods are put on the right shelf to make them cook properly. This is because hot air rises to the top of the oven by convection, and as it cools it starts to fall by convection to the bottom of the oven.

Many electric ovens are fan assisted. This means that a fan blows the hot air around the oven to make the temperature the same on all the shelves. Sometimes fan-assisted ovens cook the food very quickly, so it may be necessary to reduce the cooking time.

It is important not to open the oven door during baking as the cold, heavy air that will get drawn into the oven may cause the baked food item to sink.

ACTIVITY

1 Why is it important for the oven to be hot enough before baking cakes and scones?
2 Which part of the gas oven is the hottest? Why is this?
3 What is meant by a 'fan-assisted oven?'
4 Why is it important to keep the oven door closed when baking?
5 A cake has been baked in a gas oven and has come out with an overcooked, dark, cracked crust that has risen up to a peak.
   a) Explain why this has happened.
   b) What would you need to do to prevent this from happening again?
6 Some Yorkshire puddings have come out of the oven very flat and greasy.
   a) Explain why this has happened.
   b) What would you need to do to prevent this from happening again?
7 A roasted chicken is very well cooked on the outside, but when it is served, the inside is very pink and undercooked.
   a) Explain why this has happened.
   b) What would you need to do to prevent this from happening again?
8 Suggest a healthier cooking method for each of the following:
   a) deep fried samosa
   b) deep fried chips
   c) deep fried battered sausages

BARBECUING

Barbecuing is a method of cooking where foods are cooked on a metal grill over hot, glowing charcoal, or in a modern gas barbecue, usually outside. The food cooks by radiation from the hot coals, and if charcoal is used, it gives the food a smoky flavour. The food needs to be turned frequently to ensure even cooking. The temperature of the coals must be controlled so that the food cooks right the way through and not just on the outside. If not cooked properly, the food may cause food poisoning.

Suitable foods for barbecuing include small meat or poultry joints (chops, legs, thighs), meat products such as sausages, burgers and kebabs that contain some fat to keep them moist while cooking and fish (especially oily fish such as herring and sardines). Vegetables, such as corn on the cob, mushroom, tomatoes and potatoes, can be successfully cooked on a barbecue.

Some foods, such as vegetables, would need to be brushed with an oily dressing during cooking to prevent them from becoming dry.

ACTIVITY

1 Why does the food need to be turned frequently when barbecuing?
2 Why must the temperature of the hot coals or charcoal be carefully controlled?
3 Why do some foods need to be brushed with an oily dressing before they are barbecued?
4 How is heat transferred to food when barbecuing?

PRACTICAL ACTIVITY

Demonstrate your knowledge of methods of cooking by choosing one food commodity, such as fish, as the main ingredient. Then produce two dishes, each using a different method of cooking the main ingredient.

ASSESSMENT FOR LEARNING

Plan the menu for a summer barbecue held in the garden of a house.

Explain how you would make sure that the food was cooked thoroughly on the barbecue and would not become a food hygiene risk.

Only a few items at a time can be cooked on the barbecue, so how would you keep the cooked food hot before you served it all together?

9.3 BOILING, POACHING, SIMMERING, STEAMING, STEWING, BRAISING AND MICROWAVING

BOILING

Boiling is a method of cooking where foods are cooked in boiling water to tenderise them. When water boils, it reaches a temperature of 100°C, which causes rapid movement of the water molecules due to heat transfer by convection currents (see page 167). As the water heats and then boils, you can see the rapid movement of the water bubbles which continually rise to the top of the water. This is called a 'rolling boil', which transfers heat energy to the food by convection to cook it.

Boiling is used for many types of foods, including vegetables, whole eggs and some joints of meat such as gammon and brisket of beef.

Water soluble vitamins (vitamin C and B group) are damaged by heat and dissolve into the water. To conserve these vitamins when cooking foods such as vegetables, it is best to boil them in only a small amount of water for as little time as possible and serve them straightaway.

POACHING AND SIMMERING

Poaching and simmering are very gentle methods of cooking. Simmering is a method of cooking where foods are placed in water which is heated to just below boiling point (100°C), so that only a few bubbles rise to the surface as it is heated. For poaching, foods are placed in a small amount of water, which is heated up to just below simmering point, so there are few bubbles visible, but the water is hot enough to cook the food.

Foods such as tough cuts of meat, vegetables, pasta, rice and pulses are simmered until tender.

Foods cooked by poaching are usually high protein foods such as fish and egg-based dishes which would be damaged by higher temperatures.

STEAMING

Steaming is a gentle method of cooking, where food is cooked in the steam coming from boiling water. Heat is transferred to the food mostly by convection from the steam.

Food that is cooked in this way is very easy to eat and digest. This makes it suitable for people recovering from an illness, infants and young children, elderly people and anyone who has a health condition that affects their digestive system.

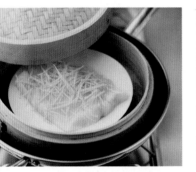

Steaming over a pan

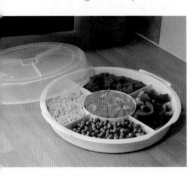

A plastic steamer

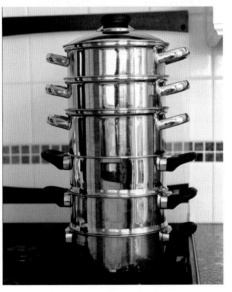

A stacking steamer

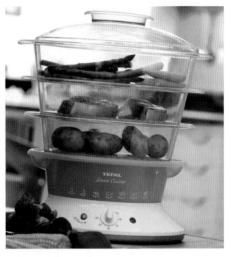

An electric steamer

Food that is cooked in this way is unlikely to be overcooked. It will have a light texture and it will not develop a hard crust.

As the food is not put directly into the water, fewer vitamins and other nutrients are lost than if the food was boiled.

Steaming can be carried out by several methods:
- putting the food on a plate over a pan of boiling water
- using a special steamer pan
- using an electric steamer
- using a plastic steamer in a microwave oven.

ACTIVITY

1 Why should vegetables be boiled for the shortest time possible in only a small amount of water?
2 How is the heat transferred to the food when boiling?
3 Why is steamed food suitable for people who are recovering from an illness?
4 Why is steaming a better method for conserving vitamins in food?

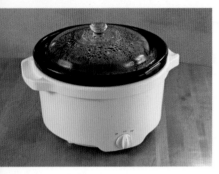

A slow cooker

STEWING

Stewing is another gentle, slow method of cooking which is suitable for foods that need to be tenderised to make them suitable to eat. This includes tough cuts of meat, poultry, hard fruits such as plums and apples, and pulses, such as beans and lentils.

Stewing is usually carried out in a covered pan on the hob or an ovenproof dish in the oven, for a period of several hours. The heat is transferred to the food through a mixture of conduction and convection.

The food to be cooked is placed in the pan or dish with a liquid (water, stock, wine) and usually other foods such as vegetables to add flavour. It is then cooked on a low heat for several hours, during which time the liquid tenderises the food and the flavour of the food develops. The liquid and other ingredients are usually served with the food as they have good flavour and retain the nutrients that have come out from the food (vitamins).

Meat that is stewed becomes very tender because the liquid and gentle heat converts the protein collagen (which makes the meat tough) into gelatine, which makes the meat tender.

Electric slow cookers are designed to cook food slowly by this method. They save on fuel, because you are not heating the whole oven, just the slow cooker, and they can be left on while you are out. The heat is controlled by a thermostat, and the liquid is held in by a well fitting lid.

BRAISING

Braising is similar to stewing, except less liquid is used. The food, usually meat, poultry or offal (e.g. heart), is placed on a bed of fried, chopped vegetables (called a mirepoix) in an ovenproof dish, and a small amount of liquid is poured over it. A lid is placed on the dish, and the meat is cooked for several hours in the oven at a low temperature to tenderise the meat in the steam rising from the liquid. Once the meat is tender, the lid is removed and the meat is browned in the oven.

Braising meat in this way can be carried out in a pan on the hob, and is usually called a pot roast.

ACTIVITY

1 Is stewing a fast or slow method of cooking?
2 Why is stewing a suitable method of cooking for tough cuts of meat?
3 How is the heat transferred to the food when stewing?
4 Why is it a good idea to serve the liquid with the food that has been stewed, such as the gravy with meat?
5 What is the difference between braising and stewing?
6 Name a food that can be braised.
7 What is a pot roast?

ACTIVITY

Make a list of foods or recipes that are suitable for the following cooking methods.
- Boiling
- Poaching
- Steaming
- Stewing
- Braising

MICROWAVING

Microwave ovens can be used to cook and heat a wide range of foods. They use relatively little electricity and so are economical to use. They also take up little space in a kitchen.

Food is cooked very quickly in a microwave oven and it takes a bit of practice to know how long to cook different foods for. It is easy to overcook foods if the wrong power setting or time is used. As the food is cooked quickly, there is less chance of nutrients, such as vitamins, being destroyed.

Most processed and manufactured foods give instructions for cooking foods in a microwave oven on their labels. This advice should be followed carefully to make sure that the food is thoroughly cooked to avoid food safety problems.

Some foods do not cook very well in a microwave oven. This includes any food that should have a crisp crust, such as pastries, breads and cakes. It is possible to buy combination microwave ovens that allow you to switch to another cooking method to finish off a dish, such as a pastry, to give it more texture and colour. Some combination microwave ovens have a grill or a convection oven that heats up to allow you to cook a wider range of foods.

Microwave ovens are a useful tool for a variety of cooking processes, such as melting butter and chocolate, making a white sauce, poaching fish and making a 'steamed' sponge pudding in a few minutes.

The food can be served in the dish it was cooked in, which saves time. Materials such as glass and most plastics and ceramics are the most suitable for use in a microwave oven – never use anything with metal in it.

Microwave ovens can also be used to defrost frozen foods, and again, the instructions must be carefully followed.

ACTIVITY

1 Name four advantages of using a microwave.
2 Name a food that does not cook well in a microwave.
3 Suggest three uses of a microwave oven when preparing and cooking food.

PRACTICAL ACTIVITY

1 Plan and cook a two-course meal (main course and dessert or starter and main course) that uses at least four different methods of cooking. Identify the methods you have used.
2 Demonstrate your knowledge of microwave cookery by planning and making a two-course meal that is totally cooked in the microwave oven.

ASSESSMENT FOR LEARNING

Look at the following recipe and identify which methods of cooking are used to prepare it.

Mixed vegetable and spinach lasagne

Ingredients:
1 tbsp olive oil
1 medium onion, chopped finely
1 clove garlic, crushed
1 aubergine (egg plant), chopped into cubes
1 yellow pepper, diced
1 courgette, diced
1 400g can chopped tomatoes
Small bunch of mixed fresh herbs, e.g. basil, thyme, coriander, parsley, chopped
200g spinach
1 egg
250g ricotta cheese
25g butter or margarine
25g plain flour
300ml milk
200g cheddar cheese, grated
1 box lasagne sheets (no pre-cooking needed)
Large shallow ovenproof dish or baking tin

Method:
1 Pre-heat oven to gas 4/180°C.
2 Heat oil in pan and add onion, garlic and fry gently until softened.
3 Add the aubergine, pepper, courgette and tomatoes.
4 Season and add the herbs. Simmer for 20 minutes.
5 Steam the spinach until softened, drain and squeeze out any water. Place in a food processor with ricotta and egg and blend until smooth. Season with black pepper and nutmeg.
6 Make the cheese sauce by melting the butter in a pan, add the flour and cook for 1 minute. Remove from heat and gradually add the milk to make a smooth liquid. Heat and stir until boiled and thickened. Add half the cheese and stir well.
7 Lightly grease a lasagne dish. Place half of the tomato mixture in the dish and add a layer of lasagne sheets. Add the spinach mixture, then lasagne sheets, then the rest of the tomato mixture. Finish with lasagne sheets.
8 Top with cheese sauce and sprinkle with remaining cheese.
9 Bake in oven for 45 to 50 minutes until golden and tender.
10 Serve with a green salad.

TOPIC 10

INGREDIENTS IN COOKING

10.1 BASIC INGREDIENTS

INTRODUCTION

In this topic you will learn about the properties and functions of some of the basic ingredients that are used in a wide variety of foods:

- fats and oils
- eggs
- sugars
- flour and other cereals
- herbs and spices.

The properties of an ingredient means:

- Its qualities – is it liquid, solid, smooth, lumpy, strong or weak?
- Its characteristics – what it can do and how it reacts in different situations such as when it is heated, cooled or mixed with other ingredients.

The functions of an ingredient means:

- What jobs it is used for in a recipe – to give colour, texture or flavour.
- The reasons it is used instead of something else.

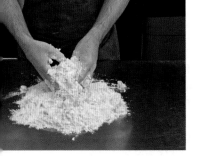

Rubbing fat into flour to make pastry

FATS AND OILS

Oils are liquid at room temperature while fats are solid at room temperature.

Oils that have been made into fats by hydrogenation (see page 42) can be made to be soft enough to spread even when they have been chilled. When heated, solid fats become liquid oils, and when they cool down, they become solid fats again. If oils are put into the refrigerator, they may become partly solid but will melt again when they warm up.

Fats and oils are used in many recipes and cooking processes.

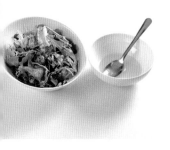

Oil used in a salad dressing

ACTIVITY

1 Describe four functions of fats in cooking.
2 Why is fat used in pastry and cake making?
3 Suggest one example of when fat is used to trap air into a mixture to help it rise.
4 Describe four functions of oils in cooking.
5 Give one example of foods that can be cooked by each of the methods below:
   a) shallow frying   b) deep frying   c) roasting

Fats: function	Reason for use	Examples
As spreads on cereal products such as bread and savoury crackers	To add flavour and to lubricate the food to make it easier to swallow	Butter, margarine and cream cheese
To make cakes, biscuits and pastries – fats are sometimes called 'shortenings'	The fat covers the flour particles with a waterproof layer, which stops the gluten in the flour from forming long strands. This makes the baked mixture have a short and melt in the mouth texture because the fat has shortened the tougher gluten strands	Shortcrust pastry, shortbread and Madeira cake
To make creams and frostings for desserts, cakes and pastries	To give flavour and texture	Butter icing, chocolate frosting, pastry cream and imitation cream
To give flavour and moisture to many recipes	The fat helps prevent water from evaporating quickly from some foods, which gives them a longer shelf-life	Foccacia bread, fruit cakes and biscuits
To trap air and make a mixture rise	Fats such as butter and margarine will trap air as tiny air bubbles when beaten with sugar	Creamed cake mixtures and all-in-one cake mixtures

Oils: function	Reason for use	Examples
For shallow frying, deep frying and stir-frying	To cook foods and give them flavour and a crisp texture	Shallow frying: eggs, bacon, fish and pancakes Deep frying: doughnuts, battered fish and meat, chicken and spring rolls Stir-frying: vegetables, strips of meat or poultry and seafood
For sautéing	To bring out the flavour of a food by allowing it to cook gently for a time	Onions: sautéing allows the sweet juices to come out of the onion, which then caramelise and make the onion turn a golden colour and have a sweet flavour
For roasting	To bake a food in oil and cause the water in the food to evaporate, which intensifies (makes stronger) the natural flavours of the food	Meat and poultry Vegetables such as potatoes, onions, sweet potato, butternut squash, aubergines and tomatoes
To make salad dressings and sauces	To add texture and flavour to other foods	Mayonnaise, vinaigrette dressing and hollandaise sauce
As dips for bread	To add flavour and texture to the bread instead of using a fat spread	Oils flavoured with herbs and garlic

EGGS

Eggs contain a lot of protein (see page 102), which will denature (change) in different processes, for example, if the raw egg is heated or whisked.

Egg yolk contains a substance called lecithin (this is how you say it: less-i-thin), which prevents oil and water from separating.

Eggs are used in many recipes and cooking processes.

Eggs: function	Reason for use	Examples
To trap air	Egg protein can stretch as it is whisked or beaten on its own or with other ingredients As it does so, it traps air as lots of tiny bubbles The trapped air adds lightness to uncooked foods such as mousses and cold soufflés, and causes baked mixtures to rise	Egg yolk and white together: whisked sponges where egg and sugar are whisked together, then flour is added; cakes where the egg is added to fat, sugar and flour and beaten to trap air Egg white: meringue, where egg whites and sugar trap air to form a stiff foam; mousses and soufflés
To bind ingredients together	Egg protein will coagulate (become solid) when it is heated. If it is mixed with other ingredients, the coagulated protein will hold them all together	Stuffing for meat and poultry, potato croquettes and fish cakes
To coat products to protect them when they are fried	Fried foods are dipped before frying in egg then breadcrumbs or in batter that contains egg. The egg protein coagulates in the hot oil and seals and protects the food inside as it cooks	Fish in batter, Scotch eggs and apple fritters
To thicken products	As egg protein is heated and coagulates, it causes other ingredients to thicken	Sauces, such as egg custard sauce (sauce Anglaise)
To prevent oil and water from separating	The lecithin in the egg yolk holds the oil and water together (this is called emulsifying) and stops them separating out	Mayonnaise: the oil and vinegar (which contains water) are prevented from separating by the egg yolk
To glaze products and give them colour and shine	The protein forms a golden brown colour with the starch or sugar in products when it is brushed on the surface and then heated	Bread rolls, scones, pies and mashed potato (on a shepherd's pie)
To enrich products	Eggs contain a wide range of nutrients (see page 102), so by adding them to other foods, the nutrients are added	Sauces, custards, mashed potato, pastry, milk puddings, stuffings and pasta
To garnish products	Sliced or quartered hard boiled eggs give colour and shape to foods	Salads

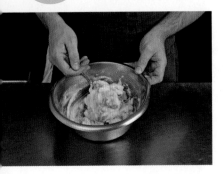

Using egg to bind a fish cake mixture

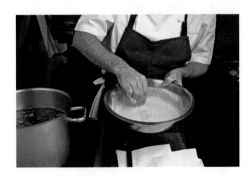

Using egg to coat food before deep frying

ACTIVITY

1 List six functions of eggs.
2 Give an example of when eggs are used to trap air.
3 Give three examples of when eggs are used to glaze a food product.
4 What is meant by coagulation?
5 What is meant by emulsifying?
6 Give an example of when eggs are used as an emulsifier.

SUGARS

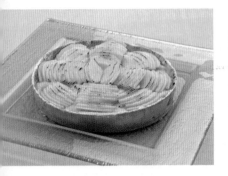

Caramelised sugar forms the topping for this apple tart

Sugar used in cooking (sucrose) is made of crystals which vary in size according to the type of sugar. Brown sugars still contain some natural impurities called molasses.

Sugars can dissolve in water and other liquids. Sugar crystals melt when heated and then form a syrup which caramelises (becomes a golden brown colour) as it is heated. It reaches very high temperatures when it is a syrup. Sugar will burn if it is overheated.

Sugar will soften gluten in baked goods such as cakes and biscuits.

Sugars are used in many recipes and cooking processes.

ACTIVITY

1 Give two functions of sugars in cooking.
2 Give two examples of when sugar is used to add texture to food.
3 Describe the effect of sugar on gluten.
4 Your friend makes a plain sponge cake and decides to add extra sugar to the recipe. Using your knowledge about the functions of sugars, describe what might happen to the cake when it is baked.
5 Give two examples of when sugar is used to trap air in a mixture.
6 What is caramelisation?
7 Give two examples of when sugar is used to give foods a golden colour.

Sugars: function	Reason for use	Examples
To add sweetness and enhance the flavour of foods such as fruits	Sugar (sucrose) can be detected by taste buds on the tongue, and humans have a natural preference for sweet foods. Sweet foods are popular and sugar is added to a variety of ready-made foods to make them more acceptable. Brown sugars add extra flavour to foods because of the molasses they contain	Chocolate and non-chocolate confectionery, biscuits, cakes, sauces, soups, soft drinks, hot drinks, desserts, yogurts, breakfast cereals, pastries, breads and bread products, gingerbread, fruit cakes
To add texture	Sugar crystals add texture to foods depending on the size of the crystals Boiled sugar is used to make confectionery (sweets and candies) Sugar softens the gluten in baked items when they are heated in the oven. This makes the product have a delicate 'crumb' texture If you add too much sugar, the gluten will be softened too much and the baked cake or biscuit will collapse	Icing sugar makes very smooth icing and confectionery Demerara sugar adds texture to foods such as flapjacks and the top of fruit cakes Toffees, caramels, boiled sweets, fudge and chews Cakes, biscuits, sponge puddings
To trap air	Sugar and egg (whisked together) or sugar and fat (butter or margarine) beaten (creamed) together will trap lots of air which will raise a baked product when it is cooked	Whisked sponges, cup cakes, all-in-one cakes and creamed sponge cakes
To add colour	Sugar will caramelise when heated and give foods a golden brown colour	Cakes, biscuits, sponges, crème caramel, toffees, fudges, caramels and buns

FLOUR (WHEAT)

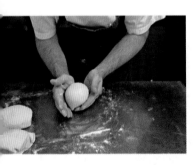

Using flour to make bread dough

Wheat flours contain the protein gluten. The amount of gluten they contain depends on the type of wheat. When gluten absorbs water, it forms very long strands and becomes very elastic and stretchy. Gluten allows doughs, such as bread dough, to rise when gas bubbles from yeast, baking powder or air (which are trapped inside the dough) start to expand with the heat of the oven. Gluten coagulates (becomes solid) when the heat is high enough, which causes the dough to set.

Wheat flours contain the carbohydrate starch. The starch is found in very small 'packets' called granules. When starch is mixed with cold water, it does not dissolve, but when the water and starch is heated up, the starch granules start to absorb the water, soften and swell. The swelling of the starch granules causes the mixture to thicken. Some of the starch granules break and release the starch which forms a gel – called gelatinisation. (The same thing happens in other starchy foods such as rice, pasta, potatoes and oats.) Starch is converted to dextrin when cooked in dry heat such as baking or grilling (toasting). This gives products such as toasted bread and the crust of cakes and biscuits a golden colour and crisp texture.

Wheat flours are used in many recipes and cooking processes as shown in the table on the next page.

Wheat flours: functions	Reason for use	Examples
Strong plain flour – produces very elastic doughs	It contains more than 10 per cent protein so makes lots of gluten strands and a very stretchy dough for products that need to rise a lot when baked	Breads, buns, choux pastry, puff pastry and batters (Yorkshire pudding)
Soft plain flour – produces weaker doughs	It contains less than 10 per cent protein, so makes a less stretchy, more tender dough that does not rise so much when baked, and can be easily 'shortened' by fat to make a 'melt-in-the-mouth' product	Shortcrust pastry, cakes and biscuits
Self-raising flour – produces weaker doughs	It contains less than 10 per cent protein, so makes a less stretchy, more tender dough that rises when baked due to the addition of baking powder. It can be easily 'shortened' by fat to make a 'melt-in-the-mouth' product	Cakes, biscuits and scones
Durum wheat flour – to make pasta dough	It contains more than 10 per cent protein, but its gluten is very tough and does not stretch very well, so is unsuitable for bread dough	Fresh pasta dough

ACTIVITY

1 Name the protein found in wheat flour.
2 Why is strong plain flour used in bread making?
3 Why is soft plain flour used in pastry making?
4 Suggest two recipes that can be made using self-raising flour.
5 Name the ingredient that is added to self-raising flour to make mixtures rise.
6 Name the type of flour that you would use for each of these recipes:
   a) bread rolls
   b) shortcrust pastry
   c) sponge cake
   d) scones
   e) shortbread biscuits
7 Explain why you have chosen each of the types of flour in question 6.

PRACTICAL ACTIVITY

Plan and cook some recipes that demonstrate how air is trapped and used to make mixtures rise. Explain how the properties of the ingredients have caused the air to be trapped.

1 Show your understanding of the properties of fats, eggs, sugars and flours, by explaining the function of each ingredient in the following recipes (the first one has been done for you to help you).

Recipe name and ingredients	Function of each ingredient
Savoury herb scones:	
Self-raising flour	Provides texture by allowing the dough to stretch when the liquid is added. The baking powder in it produces bubbles of CO_2 gas which expand in the oven heat and make the mixture rise. The starch and gluten in the flour set when baked to give texture.
Butter	Adds flavour and texture to the scones by slightly shortening the gluten strands and helping prevent water from evaporating from them.
Dried herbs	Add flavour and colour.
Milk	Adds moisture and enables the dough to form.
Eggs	Adds moisture, enriches the scone and helps the dough to set in the oven. Adds a golden colour when used as a glaze on the tops of the scones.

Chocolate sponge cake:
* Self-raising flour
* Cocoa powder
* Margarine
* Caster sugar
* Eggs

Shortbread biscuits:
* Soft plain flour
* Butter
* Caster sugar

Fruit buns:
* Strong plain flour
* Yeast
* Butter
* Egg
* Water
* Sugar
* Mixed spice
* Raisins and currants

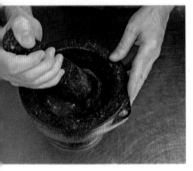

Using a pestle and mortar

HERBS AND SPICES

Herbs and spices are used in many types of cooking from different cultures and regions of the world – the Middle East, the Far East, Africa and South America.

Herbs are the leaves (and sometimes the stems, flowers and roots) of plants that contain aromatic oils which can be used to flavour foods. The oils are released from the herbs by cutting, crushing or heating.

Spices are the dried roots, seeds or barks of plants which also contain aromatic oils. They are sold as either crushed or powdered or as whole seeds. The flavourings from whole seed spices can be released by gently heating the seeds then crushing them in a pestle and mortar.

Herbs are used in many recipes and cooking processes as shown in the table on the next page.

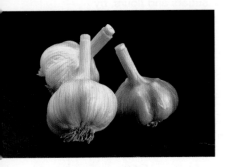

Garlic

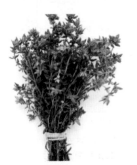

Thyme

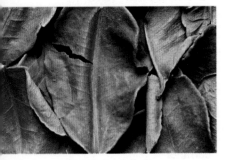

Kaffir lime leaves

Herbs: examples	Where used
Basil	In salads, with roasted vegetables, with tomatoes, pasta dishes, salad dressings and quiches
Bay leaf	In stock making, meat stews, fish dishes and soups
Chives	In salads, jacket potatoes with cheese, in cottage cheese, omelettes and soups
Coriander (cilantro)	In curries, dhals, chutneys, with fish and chicken, in stir-fries, in Middle Eastern and Far Eastern cooking and in salsas
Fennel	In Mediterranean cooking, salads and salad dressings, sauces, stuffings and fish dishes
Garlic	In stews, soups, salads, with chicken and other meats, in butter and roasted with vegetables
Kaffir lime leaves	In Thai, Malaysian and Indonesian cooking, in soups, stews and curries
Lemon balm	In fish and poultry dishes, salads, stuffings and custards for desserts
Lemon grass	In Thai cookery, curries, soups, casseroles, with chicken and seafood
Mint (there are many different types, e.g. spearmint, peppermint)	In drinks, desserts, sauces (with lamb), tea, stuffings, salads, tabbouleh (Middle Eastern salad) and raita (a cooling accompaniment to curries)
Oregano	In tomato dishes, pizzas, meat loaves, stuffings, pasta dishes and stuffed peppers
Parsley	In salads, sauces with fish, with potatoes, Italian and French cooking
Rosemary	In lamb and poultry cooking, with vegetarian dishes, stuffings and stock making
Sage	In stuffings, sausages, with chicken and Italian cooking
Thyme	In Mediterranean cooking, with tomatoes and peppers, in stuffings and pâtés, in omelettes, with poultry and meats

There are many spices that are used in many recipes and cooking processes.

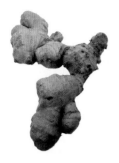

Ginger

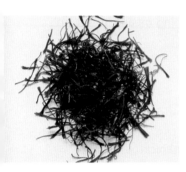

Saffron

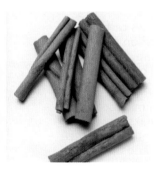

Cinnamon

Spices: examples	Where used
Anise (star anise)	Used in Chinese cooking, used in meat and poultry dishes and with fruits
Cardamom (seeds)	Used in Indian, North African, Arabic and German cooking in a variety of meat, fish and sweet dishes and drinks
Cayenne pepper (made from chilli peppers)	In cheese and egg dishes, savoury crackers, curries, fish pie, macaroni cheese
Chilli peppers (there are many different types with different strengths from mild to very hot)	In a wide variety of meat, poultry, fish and vegetable dishes Used fresh or dried whole/powdered
Cinnamon and cassia (from the bark of trees)	In cakes, biscuits, breads, buns, meat and poultry dishes, mulled wine, apple pie and confectionery
Cloves	In Chinese five spice mixture, Asian curry mixtures, with poultry, ham, fruits, in biscuits, cakes and breads
Coriander (seeds)	In Middle Eastern and South East Asian cooking, in meat and poultry dishes, chutneys, curry mixes (garam masala)
Cumin (seeds)	Often used with coriander seeds In Middle Eastern, Indian, Mexican and North African (especially Moroccan) cookery
Ginger (either fresh or powdered or preserved in syrup)	In a wide variety of meat, poultry, fish and sweet dishes from many countries Also used in pickles and chutneys and baked goods such as cakes and biscuits
Mustard (seeds)	Used in a variety of countries to flavour meat, poultry and fish dishes, as well as some baked and cheese products Made into a sauce and used in salad dressings
Nutmeg and mace	Both come from the nutmeg tree and are used in savoury and sweet dishes and drinks Nutmeg is added to cheese sauces, tomato and fish dishes, as well as cakes, breads, puddings and pastries
Paprika (powder made from mild chillies)	In Hungarian cooking (goulash), Austrian cooking, and used in Spain as smoked paprika In meat and fish dishes
Saffron (from part of a crocus flower)	Used in Italian, Spanish and French cooking, as well as in a variety of baked goods Gives a yellow colour and delicate flavour
Turmeric (fresh or powder)	Used as an ingredient in curries and curry pastes, pickles and chutneys
Vanilla (seed pod, also sold in liquid form)	Used mostly in sweet recipes for desserts, sauces, cakes, biscuits and ice creams

WHAT ARE RAISING AGENTS?

Many recipes for baked items such as cakes, biscuits, pastries and desserts have a light, spongy or flaky texture. In order for them to be like this, their mixtures have to be raised during baking. Raising agents are used to make mixtures light. Gases expand when they are heated and they can raise a mixture (bread dough, cake mixtures, pastries and batters) when it is baked. Raising agents are used to put a gas into a mixture.

Raising agents are also known as leavening agents. Leavening means 'to lift up'.

The gases used are:
- carbon dioxide (CO_2)
- air (a mixture of gases)
- steam (water as a gas).

As a mixture cooks, the expanded gas bubbles become set inside it and this gives the baked mixture a soft, spongy and light texture.

There are two groups of raising agents: chemical and mechanical.

Chemical raising agents

Baking powder is a mixture of two chemicals (an alkali and an acid), which react when there is moisture and heat, like this:

bicarbonate of soda + cream of tartar = carbon dioxide gas bubbles

Baking powder is added to plain flour to make self-raising flour, but you can buy it and add it yourself, by following the instructions on the carton as to how much to use. Once you have made a mixture with baking powder in it, you need to bake it quickly as it starts to react quickly. It is used for making scones, cakes, sponge puddings and some biscuits.

Bicarbonate of soda is also known as baking soda, and it produces carbon dioxide gas when there is moisture and heat. It can only be used on its own in strong flavoured mixtures such as gingerbread as it leaves a 'soapy' flavour in the mixture. If an acidic liquid is added to the mixture (lemon juice or buttermilk) then the soapy flavour does not happen.

Yeast is a tiny, single-celled plant that you can only see under a microscope. When it has moisture, warmth and food (sugar or starch), it breaks down the food into carbon dioxide gas and alcohol (this is called fermentation). Yeast is used to make bread and other fermented doughs such as buns and doughnuts, because the gas bubbles make the stretchy bread dough rise when it is left in a warm place for about an hour. The alcohol evaporates in the heat of the oven when the bread is baked.

Mechanical raising agents

Air is a mixture of gases and it can be put into a mixture in various ways to make it rise:
- Sieving flour and trapping air between the flour particles.
- By creaming fat (butter or margarine) and sugar together. This traps lots of tiny air bubbles which then expand and make a cake mixture rise in the oven. The bubbles are prevented from escaping from the mixture by the egg which is added and sets around the bubbles when the mixture is baked.

Baking powder gives off bubbles

Yeast fermenting

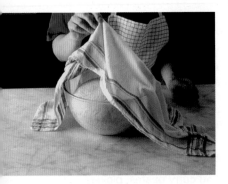

Yeast causes dough to rise

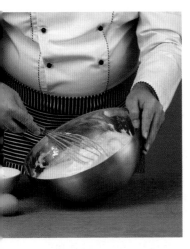

Whisking eggs and sugar

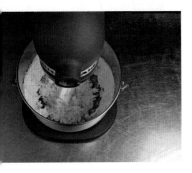

Creaming fat and sugar in a blender

- By whisking eggs or egg whites with sugar. This traps a large amount of air in the egg protein and is used as the raising agent for sponges.
- By folding and rolling a mixture such as puff pastry, where layers of air are trapped between layers of pastry. During baking, the air expands and the fat in the pastry melts. This leaves a space that is filled by steam from the water in the mixture, and also lifts the mixture.
- By rubbing in fat to flour. This traps some air in mixtures such as pastries, biscuits and cakes.

Steam is water as a gas (vapour), which is produced when water is heated. It is used as a raising agent in mixtures that contain a lot of water, such as batters, choux pastry and puff pastry. It is important that the oven temperature is hot enough to make the steam as quickly as possible inside the mixture, so that it rises properly. The oven door should not be opened while the mixture is rising, because the cold, heavy air that will go into the oven will make the rising mixture collapse.

ACTIVITY

Try to work out what has gone wrong with each of the following mixtures, by choosing one of the answers and giving a reason for your choice of answer.

1 A chocolate cake has come out of the oven very flat and heavy. This is because:
   a) That's how chocolate cakes should be.
   b) Plain flour was used instead of self-raising flour.
   c) The oven temperature was too high.
2 A Swiss roll has come out of the oven very flat and crisp and it cracks when it is rolled up. This is because:
   a) The flour was beaten into the mixture instead of folded in which knocked all the air out.
   b) The oven temperature was too high.
   c) The wrong sugar was used.
3 Some scones have risen very well in the oven, but they taste soapy and dry. This is because:
   a) Sour milk was used to mix them.
   b) The oven was not hot enough.
   c) Bicarbonate of soda on its own was used as the raising agent.
4 Some bread rolls have come out very heavy and chewy. This is because:
   a) The yeast was dead and therefore could not make carbon dioxide gas.
   b) Self-raising flour was used.
   c) The yeast was very active.
5 Some puff pastry slices have come out of the oven very greasy and flat without many puffed layers. This is because:
   a) The oven temperature was too high.
   b) The oven temperature was too cool.
   c) The wrong fat was used.

ACTIVITY

1 Name three chemical raising agents.
2 Name two mechanical raising agents.
3 Describe two ways that air can be added to mixtures.
4 Find a recipe for cupcakes. Read through the method. List all the ways that air is added to help make the cupcakes rise.
5 Name the raising agent that is used when making bread.

PRACTICAL ACTIVITY

1 Completely fill a drinking glass with flour and tap it to make sure it is really full. Sieve the flour from the glass twice on to a piece of paper. Try to put all the flour back into the glass. What do you notice? Can you explain what has happened? Why is sieving important?

2 Dissolve 1 teaspoon of dried yeast in 100mls of warm water and add 1 teaspoon of sugar. Leave in a warm place for ten minutes and write down what happens.

Repeat this four times, but instead of warm water and sugar:
a) Use cold water and sugar and leave in a cold place.
b) Use salt instead of sugar and leave in a warm place.
c) Use boiling water and sugar and leave in a warm place.
d) Use warm water only (no sugar) and leave in a warm place.

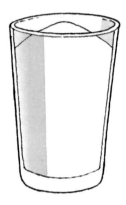
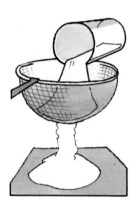
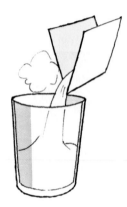

PRACTICAL ACTIVITY

Plan and make one savoury item and one sweet item that demonstrate the use of yeast.

ASSESSMENT FOR LEARNING

Test yourself or a partner.

Look at the statements below and on a piece of paper, put a tick ✓ against all the ones you can do, without looking at the textbook. If you can tick them all, well done! Make sure you can remember them in case you are asked to repeat them.

I can...

☐ Name two chemical raising agents

☐ Name two mechanical raising agents

☐ Name the raising agent in bread

☐ Explain why cake mixtures rise

☐ Give one reason why bread rolls might not rise

☐ Explain why flour should be folded very carefully into a Swiss roll mixture.

TOPIC 11
EFFECTS OF COOKING

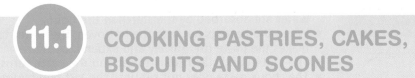

11.1 COOKING PASTRIES, CAKES, BISCUITS AND SCONES

REACTIONS TO HEAT

Breads, pastries, cakes, biscuits and scones are made from basic ingredients which include the following:

- flour (usually from wheat)
- fat (butter, margarine, oil, lard or vegetable fat)
- sugar (sucrose, honey, syrup)
- eggs
- other liquids (fruit juice, milk, water)
- raising agents (see page 188)
- flavourings (spices, herbs, cocoa, coffee)
- added ingredients (nuts, seeds, dried fruit, fresh fruit, vegetables).

When these products are baked in the oven, the ingredients react to the heat in different ways to produce the characteristic appearance, texture, colour and flavour of each product.

These are the changes that take place when each food product is baked.

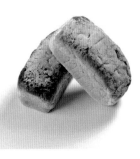

Breads and buns

In breads and buns that are leavened (raised with yeast), the changes during cooking are:

- As the dough warms up, the yeast produces CO_2 gas bubbles and alcohol.
- The gas bubbles expand in the heat and push up the dough.
- The gluten in the dough stretches.
- Water from the dough turns to steam which moves through the dough and helps to expand the gas bubbles and cook the dough.
- The alcohol vaporises and escapes from the dough.
- When the inside of the dough reaches about 68° to 80°C the gluten starts to set and the starch in the flour absorbs the water from the dough which also makes the dough set.
- The inside of the dough becomes a spongy and open network as it sets.
- The outside of the dough develops a golden crust.
- The cooked dough sounds hollow when tapped.
- As the cooked dough cools, the starch becomes firm so the bread can be sliced.
- Bun doughs cook in the same way, and the egg they contain helps the dough to set; the sugar melts and softens the gluten and the fat melts and is absorbed by the starch in the flour.

Pastries

In puff or flaky pastry:

- When the pastry dough is put into a hot oven, the fat melts and is absorbed by the starch in the flour.
- The air which is trapped between the layers of dough expands and pushes up the dough.
- The water in the dough turns to steam, which also pushes up the dough.
- The gluten and the starch set and the pastry becomes crisp and flaky.

In choux pastry:

- When the choux paste is mixed in the saucepan, the melted fat and boiling water are absorbed by the starch in the flour.
- When the paste is put into the hot oven, the water turns to steam, which makes the paste rise quickly and expand.
- The gluten and starch start to set and the paste turns a golden brown colour.
- The choux paste does not set until the last few minutes of baking, so it is important not to open the oven door and let heavy, cold air in while it is setting, which would make it collapse.

In shortcrust pastry:

- When the pastry is put into a hot oven, the fat melts and is absorbed by the starch in the flour.
- Any air that is trapped in the dough expands and makes the dough rise very slightly, but because the gluten strands are short (because they are coated in fat from the rubbing in stage) the dough cannot stretch very much at all.
- The starch and gluten both set and the pastry becomes crisp, with a 'melt-in-the-mouth' texture caused by the short gluten strands.
- The heat makes the cooked pastry have a pale golden colour.

Enriched shortcrust pastry dough cooks in the same way as ordinary shortcrust pastry, but the added sugar gives it a golden colour when it caramelises in the heat, and the added egg helps the pastry to set.

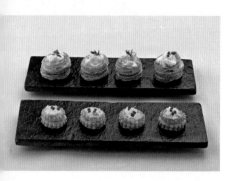

Puff pastry products

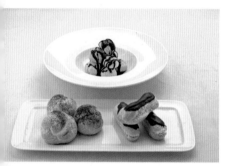

Choux pastry products

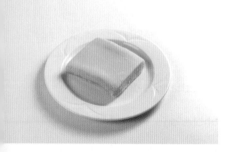

Shortcrust pastry

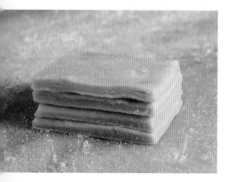

Enriched shortcrust pastry

ACTIVITY

1 Name the two substances that yeast produces as it warms up in the oven when baking bread dough.
2 What happens to the water in bread dough when it is heated in the oven?
3 What happens to the gluten?
4 What happens to the fat used in pastry making when it is heated in the oven?
5 Shortcrust pastry only rises a little in the oven. Why is this?

Cakes

In creamed sponge cakes, cakes made by the rubbing-in method and those made by the all-in-one method, these changes take place during cooking:

- When the cake is put into a hot oven, the air that is trapped in the mixture starts to expand and makes the mixture rise.
- The eggs help the mixture to set and add to the colour of the cake.
- The sugar melts and turns to a syrup, which softens the gluten to make the cake tender.
- The fat melts and is absorbed by the starch in the flour.
- The fat shortens the length of the gluten strands and makes the cake tender
- The baking powder in the flour gives off CO_2 gas, which expands with the heat and makes the mixture rise.
- The starch and the gluten in the flour set and form a fine network of bubbles which gives the cake a light, spongy texture.
- The sugar caramelises and adds colour to the cake.
- A golden crust is formed on the outside of the cake.

<table>
</table>

ACTIVITY

1 Describe what happens to each of the following cake ingredients when they are baked in a hot oven:
   a) eggs
   b) sugar
   c) fat
   d) baking powder
   e) starch and gluten in the flour

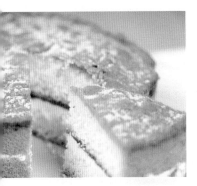

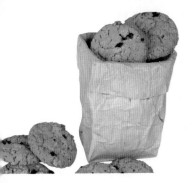

In whisked sponge cakes:

- When the cake is put into a hot oven, the air that is trapped in the mixture starts to expand and makes the mixture rise.
- The eggs help the mixture to set and add to the colour of the cake.
- The sugar melts and turns to a syrup, which softens the gluten to make the cake tender.
- The starch and the gluten in the flour set and form a fine network of bubbles which gives the cake a light, spongy texture.
- The sugar caramelises and adds colour to the cake.
- A golden crust is formed on the outside of the cake.

In cakes made using the melting method:

- When the cake is put into a hot oven, the baking powder or bicarbonate of soda in the mixture gives off CO_2 gas, which expands with the heat and makes the mixture rise.
- The eggs help the mixture to set and add to the colour of the cake.
- The sugar melts and turns to a syrup, which softens the gluten to make the cake tender.
- The fat melts and is absorbed by the starch in the flour.
- The starch and the gluten in the flour set and form a fine network of bubbles which gives the cake a light, spongy texture.
- The sugar caramelises and adds colour to the cake.
- A golden crust is formed on the outside of the cake.

Biscuits

In shortbread, the following changes take place during cooking:

- When the shortbread dough is put into a hot oven, the fat melts and is absorbed by the starch in the flour.
- Any air that is trapped in the dough expands and makes the dough rise very slightly, but because the gluten strands are short (because they are coated in fat from the rubbing-in stage) the dough cannot stretch very much at all.
- The starch and gluten both set and the shortbread becomes crisp, with a 'melt-in- the-mouth' texture caused by the short gluten strands.
- The heat gives the cooked shortbread a pale golden colour.

In cookies:

- When the cookie dough is put into a hot oven, the fat melts and is absorbed by the starch in the flour.
- Any air that is trapped in the dough expands and makes the dough rise very slightly.
- Any baking powder or bicarbonate of soda in the mixture gives off CO_2 gas, which expands with the heat and makes the mixture rise.
- The starch and gluten both set and the cookies become crisp, with a 'melt-in-the-mouth' texture caused by the short gluten strands.
- The heat makes the cookies have a pale golden colour (unless they contain cocoa)
- If chocolate chips are added to the dough, they melt and add moisture.

Scones

In sweet and savoury scones, the following changes take place during cooking:

- When the scone dough is put into a hot oven, the fat melts and is absorbed by the starch in the flour.
- The water (from the milk) turns to steam, which makes the dough rise quickly and expand.
- Any baking powder or bicarbonate of soda in the mixture gives off CO_2 gas, which expands with the heat and makes the mixture rise.
- The starch and the gluten in the flour set and form a fine network of bubbles which gives the scones a light, spongy texture.
- If sugar is used, it caramelises and adds colour and flavour to the scones.
- If cheese is added, it melts and adds to the moist texture and flavour.
- A golden crust is formed on the outside of the scones.

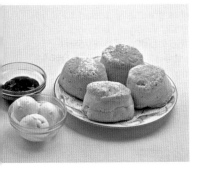

11.2 COOKING SAUCES AND BATTERS

COOKING SAUCES

Sauces are added to foods for various reasons:

- to add liquid to moisten a food
- to add flavour
- to add colour
- to bind ingredients together
- to add nutrients
- to make meals more interesting and varied.

There are various recipes for sauces and different ways of thickening sauces to give them a particular texture.

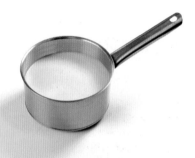

Béchamel sauce

Name of sauce	Main ingredients	What happens when it is cooked
Basic white sauce – béchamel/roux (this can also be made by the one-stage method, with all ingredients put together in a pan)	Milk Flour Fat (usually butter)	• The starch in the flour softens with the heat and absorbs the fat • The starch granules then absorb the milk as it is heated and swell • This causes the sauce to thicken • Some of the starch comes out of the granules and gelatinises (becomes 'jelly' like) which adds to the texture of the sauce
Mayonnaise	Egg yolk Salt Pepper Vinegar or lemon juice Oil	• As the oil is gradually added to the egg yolk, vinegar, salt and pepper, the lecithin in the yolk prevents the oil and vinegar from separating • As the oil is gradually whisked in, the mayonnaise thickens

Name of sauce	Main ingredients	What happens when it is cooked
Coulis (fruit sauce)	Soft fruits such as strawberries, raspberries, blackcurrants and blueberries Sugar Water Cooked vegetable puree	• The pureed fruit or vegetable gives the sauce its texture • It can be thinned out using water or thickened by heating to reduce the water content
Tomato sauce	Tomatoes Onions Celery Roasted red peppers Fresh herbs Seasoning Butter Flour Stock +/– wine or sherry	• The starch in the flour softens with the heat and absorbs the fat • The starch granules then absorb the stock as it is heated and swell • This causes the sauce to thicken • Some of the starch comes out of the granules and gelatinises which adds to the texture of the sauce • The softening of the tomatoes and vegetables adds to the texture which can either be smooth (pureed) or left with
Pesto	Fresh herbs – usually basil Garlic Pine nuts Parmesan cheese – grated Olive oil	• The pureed herbs, pine nuts, parmesan and garlic give a thickened texture to the sauce • The oil, which is slowly added, adds smoothness to the pesto
Cornflour sauce	Milk Cornflour Sugar Flavouring (vanilla)	• As the milk heats up, the starch granules in the cornflour absorb it and begin to swell • This causes the sauce to thicken as it reaches boiling point • Some of the starch comes out of the granules and gelatinises which adds to the texture of the sauce
Egg custard sauce (sauce Anglaise)	Eggs Milk Sugar Vanilla	• As the sauce starts to heat, the egg proteins start to denature (change) and coagulate (become solid) • The sauce gradually thickens until it coats the back of a spoon • The sauce must be heated gently so that the egg proteins do not coagulate too quickly, which would make the sauce 'curdle'

COOKING BATTERS

Batters are a mixture of flour, egg and liquid (usually milk). They are used to:

- make pancakes and crepes which are eaten savoury or sweet
- coat foods such as fried fish and chicken to protect the food from the high heat of the oil and give a crisp coating
- make baked items such as Yorkshire puddings and toad-in-the-hole (a baked batter with sausages)
- make fritters, which are slices of fruit or vegetables, such as mushrooms, coated in batter then fried
- make tempura (a light Japanese batter made from plain flour, cornflour, sea salt and sparkling iced water – some recipes also use egg whites) by coating vegetables and frying them in oil then dipping in a soy flavoured sauce.

When batters are cooked, the following happens:

- **Fried batters:** The egg and wheat protein sets, and the starch in the flour absorbs the liquid and cooks, which also helps the mixture to set.
- **Baked batters:** The liquid turns to steam in the hot oven and pushes up the mixture so that it rises. The egg and wheat protein sets, and the starch in the flour absorbs some of the liquid and oil it is cooked in, which also helps the mixture to set.

11.3 COOKING MEAT, POULTRY AND FISH

WHY ARE MEAT AND POULTRY COOKED?

Meat and poultry are cooked for various reasons:

- To make it safe to eat by destroying harmful bacteria that may be in it.
- To develop the flavour of the meat.
- To make it easier to chew and swallow by tenderising it.
- To make it easier to digest.

Meat (and poultry) is made of bundles of muscle fibres. Muscle fibres contain two proteins called actin and myosin. If the muscle fibres are big, the meat will tend to be tough. Meat from older animals or from parts of the animal or bird that have done a lot of work (the legs and neck) tends to be tough. Meat from younger animals and birds or parts of the animal or bird that have done little work is usually tender because the muscle fibres are small.

The muscle fibres are bound together with a substance called connective tissue. Connective tissue is made of two proteins called collagen and elastin, both of which can make meat tough if it is not cooked properly. Collagen is mostly responsible for making meat or poultry tough.

Meat and poultry also contain fat. It is found under the skin and between the bundles of muscle fibres.

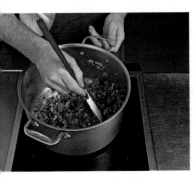

WHAT HAPPENS WHEN MEAT AND POULTRY ARE COOKED?

Before cooking, there are various methods of helping to make the meat tender before it is cooked. These include:

- scoring (cutting) muscle fibres to make them shorter
- pounding (hitting) the meat with a special hammer to break up the muscle fibres
- marinating (soaking) meat in an acid (lemon juice or vinegar) or alcohol (red wine or cider), which changes the protein structure.

The chart below explains the changes that take place when meat (and poultry) is cooked.

	Changes that happen when cooked
Texture	• As the meat is heated, the proteins in the muscle fibres (actin and myosin) denature (change) and the texture becomes firmer and the meat shrinks
	• If tough cuts of meat (from the neck or leg) are cooked slowly, with liquid (in a stew), the collagen in the connective tissue is changed to gelatine, which makes the meat tender
Flavour	• The fat between the bundles of muscle fibres melts which adds flavour (and moisture)
	• The fat under the skin melts and makes the skin become crispy if the meat is grilled, roasted or barbecued
	• As the actin and myosin denature, they squeeze out the flavoured liquid inside the muscle fibres. This liquid is called the meat extractives
	• In grilled, roasted and fried meat, these extractives come to the surface of the meat and form a sticky, brown, well flavoured substance (used to make gravy from roasted meat)
	• In stews and casseroles, the extractives go into the liquid the meat is cooking in and give it flavour
	• Meat that comes from parts of the animal that have done lots of work tend to have more flavour because the large muscle fibres contain more extractives than parts of the body that have done little work
	• Every type of meat and poultry has its own unique flavour, which is mostly due to the fat in the meat and what the animal has eaten during its life
Colour	• The colour of meat is caused by a protein called myoglobin and some haemoglobin from blood
	• Different types of muscle fibre, which do different amounts of work (meat tends to be darker in colour from parts of the animal or bird that do the most work, such as the legs, and lighter from those parts that do the least, such as the breast)
	• During cooking, the myoglobin changes to a brown colour

Changes that happen when cooked	
Nutritional value	• If meat is overcooked, it becomes dry and the proteins in it become less easy to digest • B vitamins, especially B1 (thiamin) are easily damaged by heat • Some minerals from the muscle cells are squeezed out and go into the liquid the meat is cooking in or into the pan • The fat on meat can be trimmed before cooking to reduce its energy value • If meat is grilled, the fat will run out of it, which will also reduce its energy value

WHAT HAPPENS WHEN FISH IS COOKED?

The structure of fish is similar to meat, but fish has less connective tissue so it is more tender and takes less time to cook.

White fish has very little fat in the muscle and so it must be cooked gently and for a short time to prevent it from becoming dry. The flesh becomes firm, opaque white and comes away from the bones easily in flakes when it is cooked.

Oily fish has fat in the muscle and is less likely to become dry when it is being cooked. It has a darker colour than white fish when cooked, and also comes away from the bones easily.

ACTIVITY

1 Give two reasons why meat is cooked.
2 What is myosin?
3 Name the substance that binds muscle fibres together.
4 Name the two proteins that make up connective tissue.
5 Describe two ways of making meat tender before cooking it.
6 Explain what happens to the texture and flavour of meat when it is grilled or

ASSESSMENT FOR LEARNING

1 Tougher cuts of meat tend to be less expensive than tender cuts of meat and they usually have more flavour. If they are cooked properly, they can become tender. Suggest some main meals, cooking methods and accompaniments using the following cuts of meat.

- Neck of lamb or mutton
- Shoulder of lamb
- Chicken legs
- Leg of pork – knuckle end

- Shin of beef
- Brisket of beef
- Bacon gammon hock

2 Fish is easy and quick to cook and can be made into some very tasty meals. Suggest some main meals, cooking methods and accompaniments using the following fish.

- Salmon steaks
- Whole sardines

- Mackerel fillets
- Cod steaks

11.4 COOKING VEGETABLES AND FRUIT

WAYS TO COOK VEGETABLES AND FRUIT

Many vegetables and fruits are eaten raw, which means that their flavour, texture, colour and nutritional value remain mostly unchanged. When they are cooked to alter their texture, care should be taken to preserve as much of the flavour, colour and nutritional value as possible.

There are various methods of cooking vegetables and fruits, including:

- boiling and simmering
- steaming
- stewing
- stir frying
- frying
- roasting
- baking
- microwaving.

Cooking vegetables

Different cooking methods suit different parts of plants. Parts of the plant that grow above the ground (stems, leaves, bean pods, shoots and flowers) need fairly short cooking times using the minimum amount of water – boiling, simmering, stir-frying, steaming.

Parts of the plant that grow below the ground (roots, tubers, bulbs) need longer cooking times and can better tolerate higher temperatures used in baking, roasting, frying, as well as boiling, steaming, microwaving and stir-frying.

These are the changes that take place when vegetables are cooked.

Changes in texture:

- Cooking softens the walls of cells in plant tissues, which releases the water inside the cells and makes the texture soften.
- This makes the vegetables lose a lot of bulk – leafy vegetables such as spinach lose a lot of bulk when boiled in water.
- Gradually the cells separate from each other so that the vegetables break up and become mushy.
- The starch granules in vegetables such as potatoes and carrots absorb water, soften and swell, which makes the vegetable tender and drier.

Changes in flavour:

- The flavour of vegetables is intensified when they are cooked – carrots are sweeter when they have been cooked.
- Heating causes certain natural chemicals in vegetables to be released and adds to their flavour – onions sautéed in a little butter will caramelise as the natural sugar they contain is released and changed by the heat.
- Roasting vegetables drives out water and intensifies their flavour as well as creating a characteristic roasted flavour caused by the reactions of carbohydrates to the dry heat of the oven.

Changes in colour:

- When green vegetables are first put into boiling water, they become very bright green. As heating continues, the colour changes to an olive green then to a grey/green colour, which is not so attractive. Green vegetables should be cooked in the minimum amount of water for the shortest time possible until they are just tender, in order to preserve their colour, texture, flavour and nutritional value.

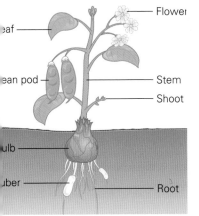

Flower

eaf

ean pod — Stem
— Shoot

ulb

ıber — Root

Parts of a plant above and below the ground

- With purple and red vegetables, such as red cabbage and red onions, the colour is easily changed by acids or alkalis in the water. Alkalis such as baking soda will turn them blue and acids such as vinegar will make them bright red (red cabbage is often cooked in water with a little vinegar added).
- Yellow and orange vegetables are usually quite stable when cooked.

Changes in nutritional value:

- Cutting and bruising vegetables causes damage to the cells inside, which releases enzymes that destroy nutrients such as vitamin C and some natural antioxidants. Exposing the cut vegetables to light and oxygen speeds up the destruction of these nutrients.
- It is best to chop vegetables just before cooking to minimise this damage
- Vitamin C and other water soluble substances leak into the cooking water, so it is best to use as little water as possible and to save the water and use it in gravy or sauces.
- Heat destroys vitamin C and other natural substances, so the least time the vegetables are heated the better.
- Cooking helps release some of the starch in vegetables and makes it easier for our bodies to use it.
- Cooking also helps our bodies make use of beta carotene and other similar substances in vegetables as it releases some of them from the plant tissues.

Cooking fruits

The information in the chart above applies to fruits also, but most fruits are eaten raw. If they are cooked to change their texture, the same rules of minimum cooking time and water would apply, in order to preserve their flavour, colour and nutritional value as much as possible.

ACTIVITY

1 Name a cooking method that is suitable for green, leafy vegetables.
2 Name a cooking method that is suitable for potatoes.
3 Describe how the texture and colour of green leafy vegetables change when they are cooked.
4 Which vitamin can be destroyed when green leafy vegetables are cooked?
5 You have been asked to show your knowledge and skills in preparing and cooking green leafy vegetables without losing too much of the vitamin C content.
   a) Describe how to prepare the vegetables to reduce the loss of vitamin C.
   b) Describe how to cook the vegetables to reduce the loss of vitamin C.

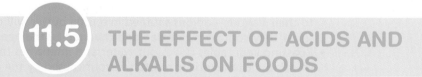

11.5   THE EFFECT OF ACIDS AND ALKALIS ON FOODS

WHAT ARE ACIDS?

Acids are chemicals that are found in some foods and other substances. Acids have a sour taste, and they give foods a sharp or zesty flavour. Here are some examples of natural acids in foods:

- Lemons contain citric acid.
- Apples contain malic acid.

RESEARCH ACTIVITY

1 Find out why dentists advise us not to drink too much concentrated fruit juice, such as orange juice.
2 Find out why meat is often marinated in an acid such as orange juice before it is cooked.

- Grapes contain tartaric acid.
- Vinegar contains ethanoic acid (old name is acetic acid).

Acids are also added to foods. For example, phosphoric acid is added to cola.

Apart from adding flavour to foods, acids also:

- help to preserve foods – because many micro-organisms cannot live in acid conditions
- act as antioxidants – vitamin C (ascorbic acid) is good for our health and also helps to keep food fresh
- enable some cooking processes to work – in jam making the fruit needs some acidity to help the jam set
- alter the texture of some foods by denaturing (changing) protein – the harmless bacteria culture added to milk to make cheese produces acids which make the proteins in the milk coagulate (become solid)
- prevent foods such as apples and bananas from going brown when they are cut.

WHAT ARE ALKALIS?

Alkalis have a soapy feel to them, and there are very few found naturally in foods. They are mainly used in toothpaste, cleaning materials and some medicines.

Bicarbonate of soda is a weak alkali which is used in baking as a raising agent, because it produces carbon dioxide gas when heated with a liquid. It is used in items such as gingerbread and scones (see page 188).

ASSESSMENT FOR LEARNING

You can demonstrate the effect of acid on protein, by making the following dessert.

Chilled lemon flan
Preparation time: 15 minutes
Serves 8 people

Ingredients:
300mls of whipping cream
1 large can of sweetened condensed milk
3 large lemons – squeeze the juice and finely grate the rind
250g plain digestive biscuits
100g butter
A flan dish – about 20cms diameter
(glass, china or metal)

Method:
1 Crush digestive biscuits and mix with melted butter.
2 Press into flan dish base, including up the sides.
3 Whip the cream until it forms soft peaks.
4 Add the condensed milk and mix thoroughly.
5 Finely grate the rind of the lemons and squeeze them.
6 Add the lemon juice and rind to the cream and condensed milk.
7 Mix together thoroughly.
8 Pour mixture into flan base.
9 Put into refrigerator to chill.
10 Serve in slices with fresh fruit.

(Variation: use two lemons and a lime)

What happens to the texture of the mixture when you add the lemon juice?

Why do you think this is?

TOPIC

12

THE FUNCTION OF ADDITIVES IN FOOD PRODUCTS

WHAT ARE FOOD ADDITIVES?

Food additives are substances that are put into processed food products by food manufacturers.

The table below shows the different types and uses of additives.

Types of additive	Reasons they are used in foods
Preservatives	• To increase the shelf-life of a food product • To prevent the growth of microorganisms (see page 207) • To prevent or slow down natural spoilage of the food (see page 205)
Colourings	• To improve the natural colour of a processed food • To change the colour of a food
Flavourings and sweeteners	• To enhance (improve) the natural flavour of a processed food • To make more varieties of a product such as potato crisps • To create new food products with unusual flavours such as sweets and drinks
Emulsifiers and stabilisers	• To make sure the food product stays stable by preventing ingredients from separating out when the product is stored • To make the food easier for a manufacturer to produce and to give it the same texture, shape and consistency each time it is made, so that customers know what to expect
Thickeners	• To improve the texture and 'mouth feel' of products such as yogurts and custards

There are three groups of additives:
- natural substances which come from foods
- additives which are the same as natural ones but have been copied and made in a laboratory
- synthetic (man-made) additives which are not found in natural foods and are made in a laboratory.

The law and food additives

Food manufacturers are only allowed to use food additives that have been approved as safe for use by the government and the European Community (EU). The ones that are approved by the EU are given an 'E' number, and have to be regularly tested to make sure they are still safe. Additives must be listed on a food label in the ingredients list so that consumers know what they are buying.

RESEARCH ACTIVITY

The chart on the next page lists some of the most commonly used additives and what they are used for. Carry out a survey of food labels and find out some examples of foods that contain these additives. (Note that there are hundreds more additives than are shown on this list. For example, there are several hundred different flavourings.)

1 Which types of foods seem to have the most additives?
2 Why do you think this is?

Name and type of food additive	E number	What job it does
Potassium sorbate	E202	Preservative
Sulphur dioxide	E220	Preservative
Carotenes	E160a	Colour (orange/yellow)
Annatto	E160b	Colour (orange/yellow)
Betanin	E162	Colour (beetroot red)
Sorbitol	E420	Sweetener
Aspartame	E951	Sweetener
Acesulfame K	E950	Sweetener
Monosodium glutamate	E621	Flavour enhancer
Lecithin	E322	Emulsifier
Xanthan gum	E415	Stabiliser
Carrageenan	E407	Stabiliser and thickener
Agar	E406	Thickener

ADDITIVES AND HEALTH

Additives are tested for safety before they are allowed to be used in foods. However, some people are concerned about the amount and mixture of additives from different processed foods that people, especially children, consume in their food on a daily basis, and the effects these may have on short and long-term health.

There have been some suggestions that certain additives are possibly linked to hyperactive behaviour in children and the development of certain types of cancer.

The best advice for people who are concerned about the use of additives is to limit the intake of processed foods and eat more natural, unprocessed plant and animal foods, and to check the labels of foods to find out what ingredients and additives are used.

ASSESSMENT FOR LEARNING

1 Here is the ingredients list from a food label for a processed food product:

Ingredients

Sugar
Water
Partially hydrogenated vegetable oil
Glucose syrup
Cocoa powder (5.2%)
Emulsifiers: E471, E491, E481, E450
Salt
Preservative: Potassium sorbate
Citric acid
Flavouring
Skimmed milk powder

Find another label for a processed food product. Identify the additives on each of the labels. Suggest whether they are being used to preserve, colour, flavour, sweeten, emulsify, stabilise or thicken the products.

ASSESSMENT FOR LEARNING

2 Match the name of the additive to the correct definition and use.

An additive which is
used to preserve foods
such as dried fruit   Aspartame

An additive which is
used to colour foods
such as margarine   Sulphur dioxide

An additive which is
used to sweeten
products such as drinks   Monosodium glutamate

An additive which is
used to enhance flavour
such as ready meals   Xanthan gum

An additive which is
used to thicken a
product such as   Carotenes
mayonnaise

TOPIC 13

FOOD SPOILAGE AND PRESERVATION

13.1 FOOD SPOILAGE

Food spoilage means changes that have taken place in a food which have made it unfit to eat. The signs of food spoilage include:

- The food has developed 'off' flavours and smells.
- There has been a change in the appearance of the food – its colour or texture.

HOW DOES FOOD SPOIL?

There are two main ways in which food spoilage happens:

- natural decay within the food
- contamination of the food by microorganisms.

All foods would eventually spoil, but there are some foods which spoil very quickly. We call these perishable foods, and they include:

- milk
- meat
- poultry
- fish and seafood
- cream
- eggs
- soft fruits such as strawberries and raspberries
- soups, sauces and gravies.

Perishable foods usually contain a lot of water and nutrients. Processed versions of these foods that have been preserved, such as long-life milk and canned fish, are perishable as soon as they are opened and must be stored properly and used up quickly.

Labelling perishable foods

Food manufacturers and retailers label perishable foods with 'use-by' dates. This is the date by which the food should be eaten to ensure that it is safe.

The food label will also give instructions about how the food should be stored (the place and the temperature) and cooked (oven temperature, microwave power setting and time) to ensure that the food is safe to eat.

Sometimes a retailer will have a 'display until' date on the food. This means that the food must be sold by that date, but it is still safe to eat until the 'use-by' date, which is normally two or three days later.

'Best before' or 'Best before end (month or year)' dates on food labels usually apply to non-perishable foods such as biscuits, crisps and breakfast cereals. The dates mean that the food will be in its best condition before those dates and afterwards will start to change in some way – the texture or flavour. This will not necessarily mean that they are unsafe to eat, but that they won't be very nice to eat.

Stocks of food in the home, a shop or a catering company should be used up in rotation. This means using up the older food that is nearest to its use-by or best-before date before using newer foods.

Natural decay

As soon as a plant food is harvested or an animal food is slaughtered or collected, changes take place inside the food which lead to it becoming spoiled.

Two main changes happen:

- **Moisture loss**: This happens in fruits and vegetables because after they are harvested, they continue to respire, which means water comes out through their leaves and skin. For example, if you leave a lettuce for a few days, its leaves will become limp and wilted and it won't be very nice to eat. This means that fruits and vegetables need to be eaten within a few days of buying them. Other foods, such as cheese and meat, lose moisture if they are not covered up in the refrigerator.
- **The action of enzymes**: Enzymes are natural chemicals found in small quantities in living things. Their job is to speed up chemical reactions. There are thousands of enzymes, and many of them are inactive until a food is harvested or slaughtered. Enzymes are proteins and they are destroyed by heat and acids. Once they are activated, they start to break down the tissues and components of a food. They also cause fruits to ripen, for example by turning starch into sugars.

ACTIVITY

1 If you cut an apple, a banana, an avocado or an aubergine in half the surface goes brown in a few minutes. This is because enzymes in the food are released and cause a reaction. The same thing happens if you bruise a fruit. The food is safe to eat but it does not look very nice.
   What could you add to the food to stop the enzymes working and prevent the brown colour appearing? Give a reason for your answer.

2 Look at the picture of the bananas below.

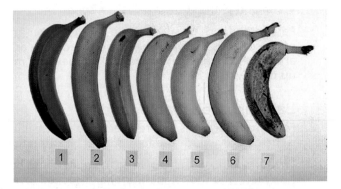

   You can see that banana number 1 looks quite different to banana number 7. This is because the enzymes in the banana have become active and have caused the banana to ripen.
   Describe what the texture and flavour of bananas number 1 and number 7 would be like. Why do you think this is?

3 When vegetables which are to be frozen, such as peas, are picked, they are blanched by plunging them into boiling water for a short time and then they are rapidly cooled.
   Why are the vegetables blanched?

ACTIVITY

1 Name two signs that indicate food spoilage.
2 Name the two ways in which foods spoil.
3 Name three perishable foods.
4 What does 'perishable' mean?
5 What are enzymes?
6 Give one example of how enzymes spoil food.
7 How are enzymes destroyed?

Contamination by microorganisms

Microorganisms are microscopic plants or animals. This means that they are very small and you can only see them under a microscope.

The main microorganisms are bacteria, moulds and yeasts. Each group has many members.

Microorganisms contaminate food (make it unfit to eat) by either producing waste products or toxins (poisons), or make it inedible just by being there. Sometimes eating contaminated food causes food poisoning.

Not all microorganisms are harmful. Yeast is used to make wine and bread, some bacteria are used to make yogurt and cheese, and some moulds are used to make cheeses.

Bacteria

Bacteria are very small – as many as one million can fit on a pin head! You cannot see them unless you look under a microscope.

They are found in lots of places, including air, water, sewage, soil, dust, plants, animals, people (especially on our hands, in our noses and mouths, and in our digestive system), food and fabrics.

Different bacteria have different shapes, as you can see in the picture on the left, which shows the bacteria under a microscope.

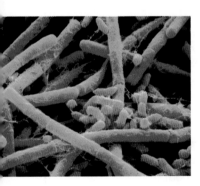

Bacteria need the right conditions to reproduce (multiply). These are:

- a suitable temperature (often warm – 37°C)
- moisture
- a food supply.

If the conditions are right for them, bacteria reproduce by dividing into two about every 20 minutes. One bacteria cell can produce millions more in the space of 24 hours. Some bacteria are harmful and cause food poisoning because they produce toxins (poisons), which make us sick (see page 218).

Bacteria grow at different rates (speeds) in different temperatures:

- At 60°C most bacteria are killed.
- At 20°C to 50°C bacteria reproduce very rapidly.
- At 10°C or lower, bacteria stop reproducing and become dormant (inactive) but they are not dead.

It is very important that refrigerators have an internal temperature of between 0 and 5°C to keep the food really cold and prevent harmful bacteria (and other microorganisms) from growing and multiplying.

Leftover foods (such as meat stew or curry) should be cooled to 0 to 5°C as quickly as possible after cooking (within 1½ hours) to prevent harmful bacteria from multiplying. They should then be used up within 24 hours and only reheated once to prevent harmful bacteria from multiplying.

High concentrations of salt, sugar or acid destroy many bacteria. These are substances often used to preserve foods.

Moulds

Moulds are tiny plants that grow on many types of foods. They are part of the fungi family, which includes mushrooms.

Moulds need the right conditions to reproduce (multiply). These are:

- a suitable temperature (often warm – 37°C)
- moisture
- a food supply.

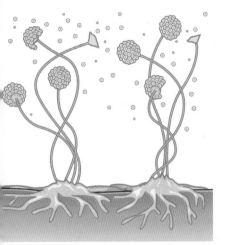

Mould growing

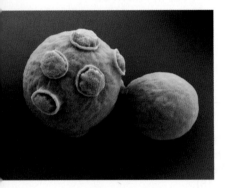

Yeast budding

They can grow at a slower rate in cold places, such as mould growing on cheese stored in a refrigerator.

Moulds reproduce (multiply) by sending out tiny air-borne spores that land on food and germinate (start to grow) if conditions are right. The germinated moulds grow a special root system into the food and break it down to extract nutrients from it.

Foods that are mouldy often look alright inside if the mould is removed, but harmful substances produced by the mould may spread into the food and be harmful to many organs of the body. So it is best to throw away mouldy food.

Mould growth is prevented by storing food in a cool, dry place, by heating the food or storing it in acid conditions.

Yeasts

Yeasts are tiny single-celled fungi. They are found in the air, soil and on the surface of fruits. Some yeasts can grow in high concentrations of sugar or acid and they can grow without oxygen.

Yeasts reproduce (multiply) by 'budding' – they send out a little bud that grows then breaks away to form another yeast cell.

Yeasts need water, warmth, a supply of food (such as sugar) and time to do this.

Yeasts are dormant (inactive) in cold conditions and they are killed at around 100°C. Yeasts can spoil jams, fruit yogurts and fruits by fermenting the sugars in them into carbon dioxide gas and alcohol (they go 'fizzy').

Did you know?

Yeasts break down sugar to produce CO_2 gas and alcohol. This is called fermentation and it is used to make bread and alcoholic drinks such as wine and beer. When bread is made, the yeasts produce CO_2 gas which makes bread dough rise, and the alcohol evaporates in the heat of the oven when the bread is baked.

Did you know?

Special harmless moulds are used to make some cheeses, such as Brie, blue Stilton and Camembert. These moulds add flavour to these foods.

A special mould called a **mycoprotein** is used to make a high protein vegetarian food called quorn.

ACTIVITY

1 Name the three types of microorganisms.
2 Name one way in which microorganisms contaminate food.
3 Give two examples of how microorganisms are used to make food products.
4 Which three conditions do bacteria need in order to grow and reproduce?
5 What effect do cold temperatures have on bacteria?
6 Which three conditions do moulds need in order to grow and reproduce?
7 Why is it a bad idea to eat foods that have been covered in mould?
8 How do moulds reproduce?
9 Which four conditions do yeasts need in order to grow and reproduce?
10 What does 'fermentation' mean?
11 What does yeast produce when it breaks down sugar?

ASSESSMENT FOR LEARNING

Here is a list of activities that should be carried out in the kitchen to help prevent food spoilage or avoid eating spoiled foods. Explain in detail why these should be done.

- Store vegetables in a cool place, wrapped or in a box and use them within a few days
- Some supermarkets sell packs of bananas where some of them are green and the others are yellow
- Wash the soil off vegetables before storing them in the refrigerator
- Wash your hands after using the toilet and before handling food
- Wear clean clothing when cooking
- Store meat and poultry in the refrigerator and use it up by the 'use by' date
- Cook foods such as chicken thoroughly
- Do not leave cooked or raw meat or fish standing in a warm kitchen
- Do not cut off mouldy parts of cheese or other foods then eat the rest of the food
- Do not eat a yogurt that has a 'blown' lid (the lid is bulging and tight)
- Regularly check the temperature of your refrigerator

 FOOD PRESERVATION AT HOME

METHODS OF PRESERVATION

Food preservation is the treatment of food to prevent or slow down spoilage by natural decay and contamination by microorganisms. Many foods are preserved, and food preservation has been carried out for many hundreds of years as a way of saving food for future use.

There are several main methods of preserving food, as shown below.

Method of preserving	How it works
Using high temperatures	• Kills many microorganisms • Stops the action of enzymes
Using cold temperatures	• Makes microorganisms inactive so they cannot grow or reproduce • Slows down chemical reactions
Drying food (dehydration)	• Kills many microorganisms by removing water from them • Prevents some chemical reactions taking place inside the food
Using acids	• Kills many microorganisms • Stops the action of enzymes
Using sugar or salt	• Kills many microorganisms by removing water from them
Controlling the atmosphere inside packaging and removing oxygen	• Stops microorganisms from growing • Stops other microorganisms from getting into the food

There are a number of methods of preservation that can be carried out in a kitchen at home.

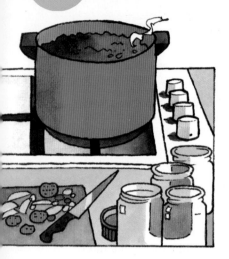

Making jam

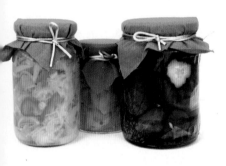

Pickles

Jam making

Jam making is a way of preserving fruit by using a combination of high temperature and sugar to destroy microorganisms (mostly yeast) and prevent any others from growing.

Fruit is stewed in water to soften it. Then a large concentration of sugar is added and the mixture is boiled to a high temperature (about 105°C). The combination of heat, sugar and pectin (a carbohydrate) in the fruit causes the jam to form a gel when it eventually cools down. The boiling jam is poured into clean, dry and heat sterilised glass jam jars, which have to be sealed while the jam is still hot to prevent other microorganisms from contaminating it. The high sugar content preserves the jam, but it can be contaminated by yeasts from the air if it is not properly made or stored.

Pickling

Pickling is a method of preserving vegetables, fruits, fish (herrings) and hard boiled eggs by using an acid to destroy microorganisms and prevent others from growing. The acid which is used is acetic acid (its new name is ethanoic acid) which is found in vinegar.

Vegetables, such as onions, red cabbage and gherkins, are prepared by peeling or chopping and are packed into clean glass jars with spices to give them flavour. Vinegar is then poured over them so that they are completely covered. The jars are then sealed and the pickles are left to mature and develop a good flavour, which takes several weeks. Good pickles should be crisp and crunchy.

Pickles, relishes and chutneys are thick, sweet sauces made from vegetables and fruits. They are cooked to high temperatures with sugar, salt and vinegar, the combination of which preserve the product and add to the flavour.

Drying

Foods such as herbs and some fruits can be dried to preserve them. Fresh herbs should be tied into bundles and dried upside down in a warm place where air circulates round them. This helps remove water from the leaves and stems and concentrates the flavour of the herbs. Once dried, the herbs should be carefully stored in glass jars with lids.

Fruits, such as apple slices, can be dried by placing them on trays in an oven set at a very low temperature for several hours, which will drive out the water.

Freezing

Many foods can be frozen in domestic deep freezers. It is very important that the temperature of the freezer is no higher than –18°C for storing frozen foods (so that the food remains in good condition), and should be between –21°C and –24°C to fast freeze fresh foods. Fast freezing is when foods are frozen very quickly in order to prevent large ice crystals from forming inside them as they would damage the texture of the food once it thawed.

Vegetables that are to be frozen should be blanched by dipping them into boiling water for a few seconds then rapidly chilling them in iced water. The blanching will stop the action of enzymes.

Frozen foods should be used within a few weeks, because even though the cold temperatures slow down chemical reactions in the food, these still take place very slowly and eventually this can affect the flavour, colour and texture.

Once frozen food is thawed (defrosted), it should be treated like fresh food as the microorganisms it contains will have remained dormant (inactive) while frozen and will start to reproduce again.

It is very important to thaw (defrost) foods thoroughly, especially foods such as chicken. This is because bacteria will remain alive in the cold centre part of the unthawed food while it is cooking, and they will start to reproduce because the food may not get hot enough right in the centre to kill them. They could then cause food poisoning.

Defrosting should be carried out in a cool place, such as the refrigerator, so that the outside temperature of the food being defrosted (such as a chicken) does not become too warm while the food is thawing. This is to prevent bacteria growing and multiplying on the food.

Bottling

Foods such as fruits and vegetables can be preserved by being placed in a special glass jar in a liquid that either contains salt (called 'brine') or sugar (called 'syrup'). The jar is then sealed tightly and the jars are heated to a high temperature for a specific time in order to sterilise (destroy harmful microorganisms) the food inside. The salt or sugar also helps to prevent the microorganisms from growing. The jars are then cooled and will remain preserved for several months as long as they are not opened.

Before they are used, the jars must be very clean and sterile and have no cracks or chips in them that could let microorganisms get inside.

Salting

The use of salt as a preservative has been known for centuries. Microorganisms cannot grow in high concentrations of salt and so it is a very effective preservative.

It is used for the preservation of foods such as cheese, sausages (especially the dried sausages that are popular in parts of Europe), fish (saltfish used in Jamaican, North African and Southern Chinese cooking and kippered herrings), and meat (beef jerky, ham, bacon, corned beef).

The salt also adds flavour which makes these food products very popular.

ACTIVITY

1 Name four methods of preserving foods.
2 How does jam making destroy micro-organisms?
3 How does pickling destroy micro-organisms?
4 What should the temperature of a domestic freezer be for storing frozen foods?
5 What is meant by fast freezing?
6 What temperature is needed to fast freeze foods?
7 Why is it necessary to fast freeze foods?
8 What does the term 'blanch' mean?
9 Name a food that can be blanched.
10 How does blanching work?
11 Why should frozen food be used within a few weeks?
12 Name two foods that can be preserved by bottling.
13 What does the word 'sterilise' mean?
14 Name two foods that are preserved by salt.

13.3 COMMERCIAL FOOD PRESERVATION

COMMERCIAL METHODS OF PRESERVING FOOD

In any average supermarket the majority of foods on sale will have had some sort of processing carried out on them to preserve them and prolong their shelf-life (the length of time they are fit to eat).

There are many commercial methods of preservation which food manufacturers' use and developments in preservation technology over the past few decades have resulted in many more types of food products being available to buy.

Using high temperatures

Pasteurisation uses high temperatures. This process is named after the scientist Louis Pasteur. It means heating food to a particular temperature for a short length of time in order to kill pathogenic microorganisms as well as some of those that cause natural food spoilage.

The process has a very small effect on the flavour and nutritional value of the food.

Examples of foods preserved by pasteurisation:

- Milk
- Ice cream
- Eggs (used by the baking industry)
- Wines
- Canned fruits
- Large cans of ham
- Fresh soups
- Fruit juices.

Sterilisation also uses high temperatures. Sterilisation uses very high temperatures to destroy all microorganisms in a food. After treatment, the food is commercially sterile.

Examples of foods preserved by sterilisation:

- Milk
- Low acid canned foods.

Ultra heat treatment (UHT) is another method. This is a method that heats a food product to a high temperature but only for a very short time, so there's not such an effect on flavour, colour and nutritional value as there is in similar sterilised products.

UHT products are often packaged in special airtight cartons made of layers of plastic and aluminium coated paperboard. When sealed, the food can be kept in the packs unopened at room temperature for about a year. This is why they are sometimes called long-life products.

Examples of foods preserved by UHT:

- Milk
- Soup
- Milk products such as cream and condensed milk
- Fruit juices
- Wine
- Sauces.

Canning, another method, is a method of preservation using hermetically (airtight) sealed metal containers that are heated to sterilise the contents inside. Metal cans are still used, but the method also includes other hermetically sealed containers such as plastic pouches, cartons and plastic trays.

The food is made commercially sterile by being heated to a high temperature after canning and sealing.

Examples of foods preserved by canning:

- Vegetables and fruits
- Ready meals
- Soups and sauces
- Sponge puddings
- Milk products and milk puddings
- Pet food
- Baby food
- Meat and meat products
- Fish and fish products
- Drinks.

Using low temperatures

Cook-chilling is a method of preserving food using low temperatures.

Cook-chilling is a method of producing ready-made foods and meals which are cooked then quickly cooled and stored at low temperatures to be heated up at home a few days later. The cold temperatures reduce the growth of microorganisms.

All types of ready-made meals, and parts of meals such as sauces, are preserved by cook-chilling.

There are various methods of commercially freezing foods. As with home freezing, the aim is to freeze the food as fast as possible in order to prevent the development of large ice crystals in the food.

Freezing method	What it means	Examples of foods preserved in this way
Fluidised bed freezing	The aim is to freeze small foods such as peas in a way that they will not stick together when they are frozen. This makes it easier to pour them out of the packet	Peas, sweetcorn and other small vegetables Berries and currants
Plate freezing	The aim is to freeze food by putting it in contact with freezing metal plates	Fish, 'boil in the bag' foods, ready meals, fish products
Air-blast freezing	The aim is to freeze the food at temperatures of –30°C to –40°C by circulating the cold air around the food	Fish, fish products, meat joints, chicken, pizzas, meals, cakes, desserts
Cryogenic freezing	Freezing food with liquid nitrogen, which has a temperature of –196°C at normal room temperature	Expensive foods such as raspberries, prawns and strawberries

Using dehydration

There are various methods of using dehydration to preserve food. Dried foods are light and take up little space, which means they are cheaper and easier to transport and store. They have a relatively long shelf-life, as long as the packaging they are stored in is not damaged, which would allow moisture and microorganisms into the food and lead to spoilage. The flavour, colour, texture and nutritional value of dried foods are affected – they lose a lot of vitamin C and some foods become tougher, such as some dried fruits and vegetables.

When dried foods are mixed with water, they become perishable and should be stored carefully and used quickly.

Dehydration method	What it means	Examples of foods preserved in this way
Roller, spray and tunnel drying	Hot air is used to remove moisture from foods	Milk, coffee, fruits and vegetables
Accelerated freeze drying	Removes moisture from frozen food by a chemical process called sublimation where the ice in the food is changed to water vapour without going through the liquid stage. Foods dried in this way reconstitute (mix with water again) very easily and are little changed in flavour or colour	Coffee, instant potato and soup mixes

Using chemicals

There are several chemical preservatives that are used in commercial preservation. These work by affecting the growth and reproduction of microorganisms, and their use is controlled by food safety laws. Some of the chemicals used are shown below.

Chemical preservative method	What it means	Examples of foods preserved in this way
Salt	Draws water out of microorganisms so that they cannot live. Salt is either added directly to the food or dissolved in water (this is called brine)	Fish, meat, cheese and vegetables
Sugar	Works in a similar way to salt, but higher concentrations of sugar are needed	Jams and other sweet spreads, candied fruit (cherries, orange peel), condensed milk, cakes and biscuits
Sodium benzoate	Stops moulds and yeasts from growing	Fruit juice, pickles and salad dressings
Sulphur dioxide	Stops the growth of some bacteria and moulds; also stops the browning effect in some foods which is caused by enzymes	Wine, beers, fruit juice, meat products and sausages
Sorbic acid	Stops the growth of moulds, yeasts and some bacteria in acidic foods	Hard cheese, bread, jam, syrups and cakes

Using fermentation

Fermentation is a natural process where specially produced harmless microorganisms turn carbohydrate into an acid, which preserves a food.

Examples of foods preserved by fermentation:

- Vinegar
- Olives
- Salami and sauerkraut
- Yogurt
- Wine and beer
- Soy sauce
- Blue cheese.

Using physical means
Physical means of preserving food take several forms as shown below.

Method of preservation	What it means	Examples of foods preserved in this way
Modified atmosphere packaging (MAP)	Changing the atmosphere around a food inside some packaging so that the growth of microorganisms is slowed down and the product can last longer MAP products are usually chilled as well	Meat and meat products, fish and fish products
Vacuum packaging	Removes oxygen which stops certain microorganisms growing, but it must be carefully controlled by chilling, as the lack of oxygen can encourage other pathogenic microorganisms to grow instead	Meat and meat products, fish and fish products, cooked vegetables, fresh pasta
Smoking	An old method of holding foods over wood smoke. The chemicals in the wood smoke add flavour but also help preserve the food, which has usually been dipped in a salt or acid solution first	Meat, fish and cheese
Irradiation	Uses radiation to fire gamma rays into a food, which kills pests, insects and some microorganisms	Onions and potatoes (to stop them sprouting), cereals and vegetables (to kill insects and parasites)

ASSESSMENT FOR LEARNING

Once food has been preserved, it must be correctly packaged and stored to maintain the quality of the food.

For each type of food in the following list, explain:

a) how it should be packaged

b) why this is important

c) how it should be stored before and after opening

d) why is this important.

- Jam
- Pasteurised fruit juice
- Frozen chicken
- Pickled onions
- Dried milk powder
- UHT milk

TOPIC

14

FOOD SAFETY

14.1 CAUSES AND EFFECTS OF FOOD POISONING

WHAT IS FOOD POISONING?

Food poisoning is an acute illness (sudden and usually fairly short) caused by eating food that is contaminated by microorganisms or poisons.

Symptoms (the effects of the illness on the body) of food poisoning are any of the following:

- nausea (feeling sick)
- vomiting (being sick)
- abdominal (stomach and intestines) pain, which can be very severe
- diarrhoea – sometimes containing blood
- high or low body temperature
- headache
- general aching of the body
- weakness and lack of energy.

In some severe types of food poisoning, a patient may have trouble breathing and swallowing and may die, but these cases are very rare.

What causes the symptoms?

Most cases of food poisoning are caused by microorganisms – usually bacteria but sometimes viruses. If the microorganisms have been allowed to grow in the food because it is not been cooked or stored properly, they can reach very high numbers and produce strong toxins (poisons) and waste products. These cause the symptoms of food poisoning when the food is eaten.

The microorganism cells, the toxins or the waste products they make can:

- irritate the lining of the gastro-intestinal tract in the body
- get into the bloodstream and other organs of the body and cause damage.

The symptoms of food poisoning can take anything from a few hours to a few days to appear and the illness can last for several days or a few weeks.

WHO'S LIKELY TO GET FOOD POISONING?

Anyone can get food poisoning, but it is especially dangerous for the following groups of people:

- babies and young children – because their immune systems (which are designed to fight disease in the body) are immature and not fully developed
- pregnant women – because the illness could affect their unborn baby
- the elderly – because their immune systems are weaker than when they were younger due to the ageing process
- people with illnesses and health conditions that weaken their immune systems, such as HIV AIDS and leukaemia, which affect their ability to fight disease.

If you have food poisoning, your illness should be reported to the environmental health department of your local authority so that they can investigate the cause, especially if you think you got it from eating food outside of your home.

In the UK there are many thousands of reported cases of food poisoning each year. However, it is thought that a lot of people become sick for a few hours after eating food but do not report it because they get better and may not realise they have had food poisoning. So many cases go unreported.

Why do people get food poisoning?
There are a number of reasons why so many people get food poisoning:

- More people eat food outside the home, which may not have been prepared hygienically.
- A lack of knowledge and understanding about how to store, prepare and cook foods in the food industry and at home, which may lead to food becoming contaminated.
- Intensive farming of food which leads to diseases spreading easily in perishable foods such as poultry and seafood.

ASSESSMENT FOR LEARNING

The graph below shows the number of reported cases of food poisoning in the UK between 1985 and 2005.

1 How many people reported having had food poisoning in:
 a) 1988?
 b) 2000?
 c) 2005?
2 A new Food Safety Act came into law in 1990, and in the following five years there were large increases in the number of reported cases of food poisoning. Why do you think this was?
3 The numbers of reported cases of food poisoning increased gradually from 1985 to 1998. Why do you think this might be? (For some clues, look at the topic on food culture on page 161)
4 Why do you think that the numbers of reported cases of food poisoning have gradually decreased since 2001?

Number of notified cases of food poisoning (UK)
Source: Health Protection Agency Centre for Infections/ Communicable Disease Surveillance Centre, Health Protection Scotland and Communicable Disease Surveillance Centre Northern Ireland

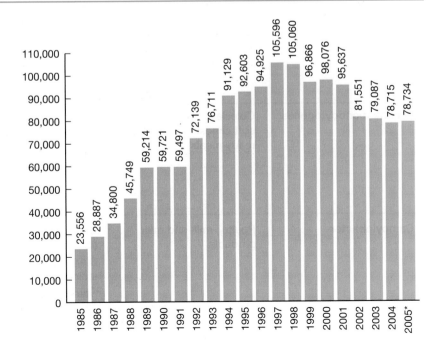

WHICH MICROORGANISMS CAUSE FOOD POISONING?

There are many types of bacteria and viruses that cause food poisoning – too many to list here. However, some of the most common ones are shown on the chart below.

Name of food poisoning bacteria	Which foods it is found in	Symptoms of food poisoning	How it gets in food
Salmonella (there are many types of salmonella, so this information is general for all of them)	Raw eggs, chicken and other poultry, meat, dairy foods, cheese, mayonnaise, sauces and salad dressings, bean sprouts and coconut	Severe abdominal pain Diarrhoea Nausea Vomiting High body temperature	Contamination from raw foods Dirty water Pests People
Staphylococcus aureus	Cooked meat and meat products, poultry, eggs, cream, salads, milk, dairy products, some dried foods	Severe abdominal pain Diarrhoea Nausea Vomiting Low body temperature Collapse	Human noses, mouths, skin, cuts and skin infections Raw (untreated) milk from infected cows or goats
Bacillus cereus	Cooked rice, herbs, spices, milk and dairy foods, meats, starchy food products, soups, custards, vegetables	Severe abdominal pain Watery diarrhoea Nausea Vomiting	Dust, soil
Escherichia coli (E.coli)	Cooked foods, water, milk, cheese, seafood, salads, meat dishes and products	Severe abdominal pain Diarrhoea Nausea Vomiting Fever	Human sewage Dirty water Raw meat
Clostridium perfringens	Meat and meat products, poultry, gravy, stews	Severe abdominal pain Diarrhoea	Sewage Soil and dust Animals Insects Raw meat
Listeria monocytogenes	Coleslaw, unpasteurised soft cheeses, cook-chill ready meals, pâté	Fever Diarrhoea Flu-like illness Blood poisoning Possible miscarriage of unborn babies	Sewage Dirty water Soil
Campylobacter	Poultry, milk and milk products	Severe and persistent abdominal pain Diarrhoea – often blood stained Nausea Headache	Wild birds Animals Pests Water Sewage

PREVENTING FOOD POISONING

It is possible to prevent food poisoning by following some simple rules:

- Store foods correctly:
  - in the correct place
  - at the correct temperature
  - for the correct time
  - in suitable containers or packaging
  - defrost food properly.
- Handle food hygienically:
  - wear clean clothing
  - wash your hands thoroughly and regularly, especially after using the toilet, handling rubbish or handling raw food
  - use clean equipment
  - do not allow raw food to come into contact with cooked food
  - do not cough, sneeze, spit over food or touch your nose when handling it
  - do not let animals or pests contaminate it.
- Cook food properly and thoroughly:
  - to the right temperature
  - for the right time
  - keep it hot before serving
  - cool leftover food quickly
  - use leftover food within 24 hours and reheat it only once.
- Clean properly:
  - clean regularly as you prepare and cook
  - clear away rubbish regularly
  - use clean dishcloths and drying up cloths
  - clean equipment properly in hot soapy water, then rinse and dry thoroughly
  - keep food cupboards and refrigerators clean
  - keep pests out of the kitchen.

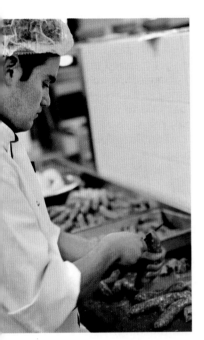

Handling food hygienically

ACTIVITY

1 What is food poisoning?
2 Describe two symptoms of food poisoning.
3 What causes food poisoning?
4 Name two groups of people who are more at risk from food poisoning.
5 Explain why the two groups you have chosen are at risk.
6 Name one microorganism that causes food poisoning.
7 Name two foods that the microorganism is found in.
8 Suggest three ways in which food poisoning can be prevented.

14.2 FOOD CONTAMINATION

Contamination means to allow unwanted substances (contaminants) to get into foods, which would make it unfit to eat. Food contaminants include things such as:

- microorganisms (see page 218)
- hair, finger nails (real ones and false ones) and nail varnish – these can fall into food and can also pass on bacteria to food because they get trapped under finger nails
- skin infections and cuts, which can contain microorganisms
- jewellery – this can fall into food and can also pass on bacteria to food because small bits of food can become stuck in decorative parts of rings
- mucus from the nose and saliva from the mouth – this can get into food from coughing, spitting, sneezing, touching or picking the nose
- dirt and dust
- dirty water
- chemicals including cleaning fluids and powders, poisonous pesticide sprays, powders and liquids
- pets and pests – this includes flies and other insects, rats, mice and birds, which can put droppings, feathers, fur and eggs into food
- small objects such as pieces of glass, metal or plastic which can fall into foods.

Cross-contamination means allowing microorganisms to transfer from one food (usually raw) to another food either by:

- **direct contact:** between the two foods (storing a raw food such as chicken right next to a cooked food such as ham, so that they are touching)
- **drips:** from a raw food falling on to another food (from a raw chicken that is been placed on a shelf in the refrigerator and drips on to foods below)
- **indirect contact:** where the microorganisms have been transferred by the hands, a dishcloth or a piece of equipment that is been used for both foods (e.g. chopping boards).

REDUCING AND AVOIDING FOOD CONTAMINATION

It is possible to avoid food contamination when preparing food in the kitchen at home by following some simple rules and practices. Many of these are common sense but it is worth stating what they are to help you understand why they are necessary.

These are set out on the next page in groups under these headings:

- food storage
- food preparation
- cooking food
- serving food
- clearing up.

Rule or practice	How to follow it
Food storage	
Follow manufacturer's instructions for storing foods	Look at the packaging and labels for storage conditions, temperatures, 'use by' and 'best before' dates (see page 205)
Store fresh perishable foods in a refrigerator that is set at the right temperature	A refrigerator should have an internal temperature of between 0 and 5°C (see page 207)
Store frozen perishable foods in a freezer that is set at the right temperature	A freezer should have an internal temperature of at least −18°C (see page 210)
Store dry goods in sealed containers in a cool, ventilated cupboard	Keep dry foods away from any moisture and contamination from dust, dirt, pets and pests
Rotate the stock of foods	Use up old foods first before opening new ones (see page 205)
Store leftover foods in suitable containers in a cold place and use them up within 24 to 48 hours	• Label the foods with the date they were made • Only reheat leftover foods once and make sure they are heated right through (see page 207)
In a refrigerator store raw foods on the shelves underneath cooked foods	Store raw foods on trays, plates or in covered containers
In a refrigerator store salad ingredients and vegetables in a special box away from other foods	Wash the dirt off vegetables
Thaw frozen foods thoroughly before cooking them	Thaw frozen foods such as chicken on a tray, in a refrigerator for several hours, not at room temperature or in warm water (see page 210)
Store food in a suitable cupboard	• Keep food away from heat • Make sure the cupboard is free from pests • Make sure the cupboard isn't damp • Do not store food on the floor unless it is in sealed containers
Food preparation	

Have clean hands	• Wash your hands:
	  – before cooking
	  – after using the toilet
	  – after handling raw meats, fish, dirty vegetables and eggs
	• Keep your finger nails short and clean
	• Do not wear false nails or nail varnish
	• Do not wear rings

Cover up any cuts, sores or infections on your hands or fingers	• Wear a blue food grade plaster • Wear a disposable plastic glove • Wear an apron or other clean covering • Wash the apron regularly • Do not wear jewellery that could fall in the food
Do not let your hair fall into the food	Keep your hair tied back or wear a hat
Do not contaminate the food from your nose or mouth	• Do not cough, sneeze or spit over food • Do not pick your nose while preparing food • Do not smoke while preparing food
Use clean equipment	• Wash up regularly • Do not use the same equipment for raw and cooked foods – wash it up in between

Rule or practice	How to follow it
Clear as you go	<ul><li>Throw away rubbish regularly</li><li>Clear the work surface</li><li>Wipe up spills and mess</li><li>Wash up between preparing raw food and cooked food</li></ul>
Keep food covered and cool needed	<ul><li>Keep perishable food in the refrigerator until</li><li>Cover foods, especially in the summer</li></ul>
Cooking food	
Cook perishable foods thoroughly	<ul><li>Make sure foods are cooked right through</li><li>Cook foods to at least 70°C for two minutes in the centre – this is called 'piping hot'</li><li>Keep food hot to at least 63°C</li><li>Use a digital temperature probe if you are unsure about the temperature</li></ul>
Serving food	
Serve food hot	<ul><li>Serve food as soon as possible after it is cooked</li><li>If it has to be kept hot, do not let it drop below 63°C</li></ul>

ACTIVITY

Design a poster for your food area at school about either preparing or cooking and serving food safely.

THE ROLE OF FOOD MARKETING AND ADVERTISING

THE FOOD INDUSTRY

In the UK the food industry is the largest manufacturing organisation, with about 500,000 people employed in the manufacture of food.

People have to eat, and depending on their individual circumstances and how much money they have and what they need to spend on their living expenses (rent or mortgage, heating and lighting, travelling), they either spend more or less on food and drinks throughout the year.

Much of the food industry is owned by a few large companies. They spend a huge amount of money each year on marketing and advertising their food products and generally make large profits from selling their products in the UK and throughout the world.

WHAT IS MARKETING?

In the food industry, marketing is the process of identifying consumers' food needs and wants and supplying them efficiently with a suitable range of food products so that the consumers are happy and the company makes a profit.

Marketing includes such activities as:

- **Market research**: finding out what the consumer needs and wants, finding out what products other rival food companies are producing and identifying target groups of people who would buy a food product.
- **Product development**: Making new products and testing their popularity and acceptability, changing existing products to improve them and extending a range of products (new flavours, reduced fat or sugar).
- **Company positioning**: Letting customers know where your company stands on different issues to do with food such as animal welfare, fair trade, environmental sustainability, diet and health, buying local foods and the use of food additives.

WHAT IS ADVERTISING?

Advertising is the methods a company uses to promote its food products. It includes activities such as:

- **Product launches**: Special introductory price, buy one get one free, free samples, money-off vouchers, tasting sessions in shops.
- **Image and brand building**: Visual advertisements on television and the internet, at exhibitions, in the streets, on leaflets and magazine and newspaper advertisements, in cinemas and shops, text messaging. Audio advertisements on the radio, telemarketing (on the telephone). The use of celebrities to promote a product.

ACTIVITY

How might a supermarket try to increase the sales of a new healthy eating range of foods?

ACTIVITY

As a class, collect some food advertisements from magazines and newspapers.

Carry out some consumer or class research to find out which are the most popular advertisements and why people like them.

Design your own advertisement for a food product of your choice. Display it to the class with everyone else's and carry out a class vote on the one that is the most appealing.

TOPIC

16

PURCHASING (BUYING) FOODS

WHAT MAKES PEOPLE BUY CERTAIN FOODS?

People are influenced by a number of issues when they buy food or any other goods. Good market research should be able to identify these issues and use them to develop food products that will sell.

The issues that influence what people buy include:

- the price of a food product
- how familiar they are with a food product
- the reputation of a supermarket, shop or market stallholder
- the reputation of a food manufacturing company
- the availability of a food product
- the reliability and reputation of a food product
- how the food product fits in with their lifestyle and status
- the amount of time people have to spend going shopping for food.

Shopping trends

Shopping habits have changed over the years as people's lifestyles and technology have also changed and developed. Some of the changes and developments in shopping for food are the following:

- The closure of many individual specialist food shops such as bakers, butchers, fishmongers, greengrocers and delicatessens in town centres (although there has recently been increased interest in specialist shops and markets, which has been encouraged by food programmes on the television).
- The sale of food and household goods all under one roof, in large, out-of-town supermarkets (superstores), which need transport to get to and from.
- The purchase of food weekly (or longer) from supermarkets, rather than daily from local shops.
- The bar-coding of food products makes it quicker to purchase foods at the checkout.
- Online ordering of food from supermarkets and other companies for home delivery.
- The purchase of foods which have travelled large distances (a lot from other countries) from where they were produced to the shop they are bought in (this is called 'food miles').
- The purchase of many convenience foods, especially ready-made meals and ready prepared ingredients.
- The use of much more packaging materials in food products, especially plastics, which use up non-renewable energy resources and has environmental implications for their disposal.

Why have shopping trends changed?

There are several reasons why shopping trends have changed, most of which are to do with general changes in society:

- More women work outside the home and therefore have less time to shop and cook.
- More people own cars and therefore are able to drive out of town to large supermarkets.
- There is a need to have many things instantly available because people live such busy lives.
- There are more opportunities for many people to travel and try out new foods in other regions and countries.

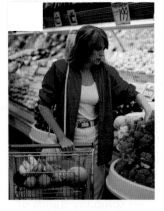

Supermarket shopping today

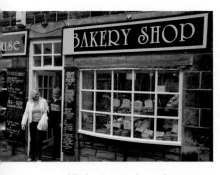

High street shopping

- Technological changes, especially computer technology, make it possible to buy foods and other goods without even having to visit a shop.
- The influence of cookery programmes and food advertising on television has encouraged people to want to try new foods.
- There has been a gradual decline in the number of people who have confidence in choosing ingredients and preparing food and know how to cook.

ACTIVITY

Here are some statistics on people's food shopping and eating habits in the UK, taken from the book *Bad Food Britain – how a nation ruined its appetite* by Joanna Blythman (published by Fourth Estate, 2006).

- 25 per cent of British households do not have a table at which they eat a meal.
- In 2003 people in the UK ate more ready-made meals than the rest of Europe put together.
- 40 per cent of food that is bought from shops is never eaten.
- People in the UK eat more than half (51 per cent) of all the potato crisps and savoury snack foods eaten in Europe.
- One person in every three people in the UK say they do not eat vegetables because they take too much effort to prepare.

1 In which year did people in the UK eat more ready meals than all of the rest of Europe?
2 How many people in the UK have a table at which they eat meals?
3 What does statistic number 1 tell you about people's eating habits?
4 How much food bought from shops is wasted?
5 What does statistic number 3 tell you about people's food shopping habits?
6 Why do you think people in the UK eat more ready meals than in Europe?
7 Why do you think people in the UK eat so many snack foods?
8 What does statistic number 5 tell you about people's cooking and eating habits?

ACTIVITY

In the table on the next page are some statistics from a publication called 'Family Food in 2007', which is produced by the UK Statistics Authority and the Department for Environment, Food and Rural Affairs (Defra), both UK government bodies.

The statistics give details of what food people buy and the trends for this between 2004 and 2007.

1 Which types of milk were sold the most in 2007?
2 What is the percentage drop in the amount of fat reduced and low fat spreads bought?
3 What is the percentage increase in the amount of fruits and vegetables bought?
4 What is the percentage drop in the amount of white bread bought between 2004 and 2007?
5 What was the average amount of money spent per person on food eaten outside the home in 2007?
6 Why do you think more people are eating fruits and vegetables?
7 Why do you think less whole milk is being bought?
8 Why do you think less processed fat reduced and low fat spreads are being bought?
9 Why do you think less processed meat and meat products are being bought?
10 Why do you think people spend nearly half as much on food and drinks eaten outside the home as they do on food and drinks eaten at home?

Food	What the statistics show
Milk	• Purchases of whole milk have fallen • Purchases of semi-skimmed and skimmed milks have gone up • In 2007 73 per cent of all milk bought was semi-skimmed or skimmed
Fats	• Since 2004 there has been an 18 per cent increase in the amount of natural fats (such as butter) bought • Since 2004 there has been a 22 per cent drop in the amount of processed reduced fat and low fat margarine type spreads bought
Fruit and vegetables	• There has been a 6.5 per cent increase in the amount of fruits and vegetables bought • The more income people have, the more fruits and vegetables they are likely to buy
Bread	• In 2004 51 per cent of all bread bought was white • In 2007 45 per cent of all bread bought was white
Soft drinks (carbonated, fizzy sweet drinks – not fruit juices)	• There has been a 15 per cent drop in the amount of non-diet versions of soft drinks bought
Processed meat and meat products	• There has been a 3.1 per cent drop in the amount of processed meat and meat products bought
All food and drink	• In 2007 the average amount of money per person spent on food and drinks eaten in the home was £24.95 • In 2007 the average amount of money per person spent on food and drinks eaten outside of the home was £11.37

Source: based on UK Statistics Authority and Defra, 'Family Food in 2007'

ACTIVITY

List some advantages and disadvantages of buying foods from these different places. Consider issues such as cost, customer service and advice about foods, ease of buying the food and so on. Give reasons for your answers.
- Supermarket
- Specialist shop – baker, butcher, fishmonger, greengrocer (fruits and vegetables)
- Online shopping
- Street market
- Farmer's market or direct from a farm

TOPIC 17

FOOD LABELLING

WHAT INFORMATION SHOULD BE ON FOOD LABELS?

When we buy our food, we use a lot of visual information, such as colour and shape to help us choose. Food manufacturers know this, and so they spend a lot of money designing food packaging and labels so that consumers are attracted to them and not to products from another company.

The packaging must not only be attractive, but it must also give the consumer information that they can use to make a decision about whether or not to buy. Some of the information that appears on food labels has to be included by law, under the Food Labelling Regulations 1996.

The following information must appear by law on a food label for most foods:

- the name of the food
- the name and address of the manufacturer, packer or seller of the food
- the country of origin – where the food or some of the ingredients in it came from
- instructions about how to use or cook the food, if appropriate (how long to cook a meat pie, at what temperature or microwave oven power setting)
- a list of ingredients in the food (in descending order of amount – the most first)
- the quantity of certain ingredients (e.g. the percentage amount of meat in sausages)
- the shelf-life of the food shown by a use-by or best before date (see page 205)
- how to store the food – where the food should be stored such as in a cool, dry place. If it is to be kept cold, additional information should be shown.

These are the star ratings for food to be stored in refrigerators and freezers:

* –6°C: 1 week (pre-frozen food only)
** –12°C: 1 month (pre-frozen food only)
*** –18°C: 3 months (pre-frozen food only)
**** –18°C or colder: 6 months (pre-frozen food and can also be used to freeze fresh food from room temperature).

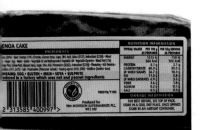

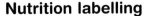

Nutrition labelling

Under the Food Labelling Regulations 1996 and the EC Nutrition Labelling Directive, guidance is given about how nutrition information should appear on food labels if it is given.

Nutrition labelling is only compulsory on foods where a claim has been made about the nutritional value, such as 'high in fibre' or 'low in fat'.

These are the guidelines that should be followed when giving nutrition information.

The following nutrients should be shown as amounts in every 100g or 100mls of a food:

- energy as kj and kcal
- protein in grams (g)
- carbohydrate in grams of which sugars should be shown in grams
- fat in grams of which saturates should be shown in grams
- fibre in grams
- sodium in grams.

The following nutrients can also be shown on the label. They must be shown if a claim is made about them:

- sugars
- polyols
- starch
- mono-unsaturates
- polyunsaturates
- cholesterol
- vitamins in milligrams or micrograms
- minerals in milligrams or micrograms.

The nutritional information should either be set out in a table or written out as a list (not both together). This is to help make the information easy for consumers to read.

The Food Standards Agency (FSA) has tried to make the nutritional information easier for consumers to understand, so that they can see at a glance whether a food is high or low in certain nutrients. The FSA has produced a 'traffic light' system of food labelling to help consumers, which shows how much of each nutrient is provided by each serving of the food:

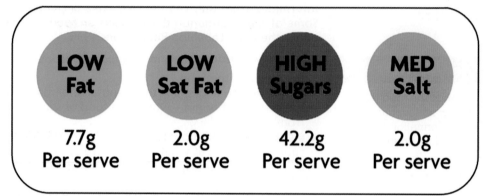

Source: Food Standards Agency

ACTIVITY

Here is a food label for Shredded Wheat.

Typical values	Per 45g serving (2 biscuits) with 125mls semi-skimmed milk	Per 100g
Energy	918kj	1442kJ
	217kcal	340kcal
Protein	9.6g	11.6g
Carbohydrate	37.5g	67.8g
of which: sugars	6.3g	0.9g
Fat	3.2g	2.5g
of which: saturates	1.4g	0.5g
Fibre	5.3g	11.8g
Sodium	Trace	Trace
Salt equivalent	0.2g	Trace

1 How many kcals will a 150g serving provide?
2 What percentage of protein does Shredded Wheat provide?
3 How many grams of sugar will a 200g serving provide?
4 How much fat will half a 45g serving provide?

Source: www.cerealpartners.co.uk

Other information that appears on food labels

Food manufacturers also put other symbols on food labels to help consumers make choices about what to buy.

Earlier in this unit, we saw an example of gluten-free labelling (page 149). A gluten-free symbol means that the food does not contain gluten (the protein found in wheat and some other cereals). People who have coeliac disease would find this information very useful.

We also saw the Vegetarian Society symbol that means that the food is suitable for vegetarians (page 147).

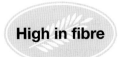

This symbol indicates that the food contains plenty of fibre which would be useful for someone with an intestinal health condition.

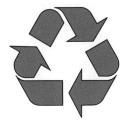

International symbol for recycling, which would tell consumers if the packaging used for the food they are buying is able to be recycled.

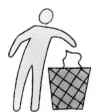

International symbol to remind people not to drop litter on the ground.

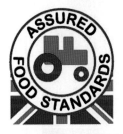

The Red Tractor logo is an independent mark of quality that guarantees to the consumer that food has been produced to high standards of food safety and hygiene, animal welfare and environmental protection. The Union flag in the Red Tractor logo provides an independent consumer guarantee that the product has come from a UK farm.

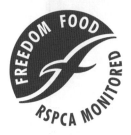

Certification Mark

The Freedom Food mark is a registered certification mark in the United Kingdom which indicates that the food has been produced to higher animal welfare standards and supported by the Royal Society for the Prevention of Cruelty to Animals.

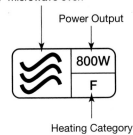

Indicates the oven is a "microwave oven"

Power Output

800W

F

Heating Category

Microwave oven symbol showing that food can be cooked in a microwave oven and at what power.

WHY IS FOOD LABELLING IMPORTANT?

The aim of food labelling is to give consumers details about a food product so that they can make an informed choice about which product to buy. This means that they can make their decision based on the information the label gives them.

The information on the label is particularly important if the consumer:

- has a particular health condition and needs to know the fat, sugar, salt or fibre content of the food
- has a food allergy and needs to know if the product is safe for them to eat
- has to make a complaint about the product (say because it is stale or has a piece of metal in it) and needs to contact the manufacturer
- has a religious or cultural reason to avoid certain foods or ingredients and needs to know if the food contains any
- has limited knowledge about how to cook and needs to know how to prepare and heat the food
- has limited knowledge about how to keep food safe to eat and needs to know the correct storage conditions for the food
- has concerns about animal welfare and environmental issues and wants to know how and where the food was produced (organically, intensively, free-range).

ASSESSMENT FOR LEARNING

1 What type of consumer do the symbols on the label indicate this food product is suitable for?
2 How should the food product be stored?
3 How can the food product be prepared for eating?
4 Is the packaging able to be recycled?
5 Can a person with coeliac disease eat this product?

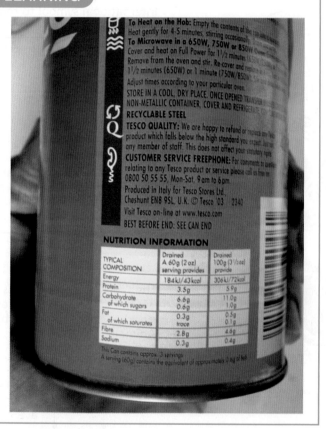

TOPIC

18

FOOD SAFETY AND THE LAW

THE FOOD HYGIENE (ENGLAND) REGULATIONS 2006

There are laws to protect consumers when they buy food to try to make sure that only good quality food is sold and that the health of consumers is not put at risk.

The Food Hygiene (England) Regulations 2006 are the most recent regulations and they cover all sectors (parts) of the food industry:

- **Food production** – farming, market gardening, fishing
- **Food processing** – factories, slaughterhouses, processing plants, bakeries, butchers, restaurants, cafes, canteens, roadside snack bars, self-employed small home businesses, burger bars, public houses, passenger ships, aircraft
- **Food storage** – refrigeration units, warehouses, shipping companies, shops
- **Food distribution** – transport businesses, warehouses, shipping companies, local delivery vans, ice cream or fish and chip vendors
- **Food retail** – shops, markets, supermarkets, hypermarkets, mail order companies, farm shops, farmers markets, non-profit-making organisations (charities), restaurants, cafes, bars, pubs, self-employed caterers, school or community functions, snack and sandwich delivery services.

These regulations extended, updated and replaced the Food Safety Act 1990 and the Food Safety (General Food Hygiene) Regulations 1995. They cover:

- food
- sources of food (crops, animals)
- drinks
- slimming aids
- food supplements such as vitamin pills
- water used in the food industry (but not the water supply, which is governed by separate legislation)
- what comes into contact with food, such as packaging, cling film, machinery and cooking utensils
- sale of food at fundraising events.

The regulations make it an offence to:

- sell food which does not meet food safety requirements – food that could make people ill because it is infected with microorganisms (the Act does not cover allergic reactions to food ingredients, although many retailers and manufacturers will now label food that contains nuts to warn people who are allergic)
- sell food that is unfit to eat, for example because it contained a dead animal, a piece of glass, antibiotic residues
- deliberately make food harmful by adding to it or removing something
- sell food which is 'not of the nature, substance or quality demanded by the purchaser' (the food must be exactly as described and of a good quality)
- mislead consumers deliberately by giving a false or exaggerated description of the food, such as picturing a gateau decorated with lots of strawberries on the packet, when the actual item inside has only one or two strawberries on it.

The regulations are enforced by:

- central government
- local government (local authorities) – environmental health department and trading standards department
- trading standards officers who deal with food labelling, composition and chemical contamination

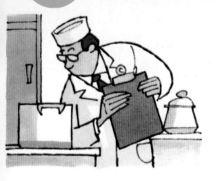

An environmental health officer

- environmental health officers who inspect food businesses and deal with food hygiene, food poisoning, contamination by microorganisms and food that is unfit for human consumption. They can close down food businesses if they break the law.

The regulations also require food businesses to:

- register with the local authority so that they can be inspected
- train the people who are responsible for handling the food in food hygiene
- follow careful procedures for storing, preparing and serving food and keep records (the temperature of refrigerators and cooked foods) to show that these have been followed correctly
- make sure that people who handle food follow basic hygiene rules.

Here are some basic hygiene rules:

1 Always wash your hands before handling food and after using the toilet.
2 Tell your boss at once of any skin, nose, throat or digestive or bowel trouble.
3 Ensure cuts and sores are covered with waterproof dressings.
4 Keep yourself clean and wear clean clothing. Do not allow loose hair to dangle or drop into food.
5 Do not smoke in a food room. It is illegal and dangerous.
6 Never cough or sneeze over food.
7 Clean as you go. Keep all equipment and surfaces clean. Use very hot water and clean dishcloths and tea towels for washing and drying equipment and surfaces.
8 Prepare raw and cooked food in separate areas with separate equipment.
9 Keep food covered and either refrigerated or piping hot (at least 70°C in the centre of the food).
10 Foods kept in storage cupboards should be properly sealed and used in rotation, following the manufacturer's guide to the shelf-life of each product.
11 Keep your hands off food as far as possible – use disposable gloves to handle foods where appropriate.
12 Ensure waste food is disposed of properly. Keep the lid on the dustbin (which should be located outside the kitchen) and wash your hands after using it. Kitchen bins should be regularly cleaned and disinfected.
13 Tell your supervisor if you cannot follow the rules.
14 Do not break the law.

All food businesses have a legal duty to protect the health of their customers and must show 'due diligence' in their everyday activities. This means they must prove that they have done everything they can to make sure that food is safe for people to eat. To make sure this is done, the regulations require food businesses to identify and control potential (things that could happen) food hazards.

To do this, they must:

- make sure food is supplied or sold in a hygienic way
- identify food safety hazards
- know which steps in the activities of the food business are critical for food safety
- ensure safety controls are in place, maintained and reviewed.

ACTIVITY

1 Name two sectors of the food industry covered by the 2006 Food Safety Regulations.
2 Name two organisations which enforce the regulations.
3 Describe the role of an environmental health officer in ensuring that food is safe to eat.
4 Describe four basic hygiene rules that food handlers must follow.

You are a regular customer in a supermarket. Make a list of the qualities you would look for and expect to see in a perishable food section of the supermarket (the delicatessen counter where they serve cold meats, pâtés and cheeses, the fresh fish or meat counter or the fresh salad bar). Do this using the following headings:

- the staff
- the equipment used to display, prepare (cut or slice) and serve the food
- the serving area (floor, walls, display shelves, counters, sink).

OTHER LAWS TO PROTECT CONSUMERS

There are other laws to protect consumers from bad practices in the food industry. These include misleading customers about what they are buying, incorrectly describing foods for sale and refusing to compensate a customer when a food is faulty. The actual Acts are:

- Trade Descriptions Act 1968
- Sale of Goods and Services Act 1982
- Sale and Supply of Goods Act 1994
- The Sale and Supply of Goods to Consumers Regulations 2002.

HOW TO MAKE A COMPLAINT

If you think there is something wrong with, for example, the food you have ordered in a restaurant, you should ask to speak to the manager. Explain calmly and clearly why you are complaining.

If you are not satisfied with how the manager deals with your complaint, report your concerns to your local Trading Standards or Environmental Health officer. They will investigate the problem if they think you have a genuine complaint.

TOPIC

19

TYPES OF QUESTIONS

For the final part of your GCSE course, you will be required to take a **written examination** to test your knowledge about what you have learned during the course.

The examination will test you on the following units of learning:

1 **Nutrition and health**
 • Function and role of the nutrients
 • The relationship between diet and health
 • Energy and food

2 **Food commodities**
 • The nutritional value and types of food commodities (meat, fish, eggs, dairy foods, fruit, vegetables, cereals, sugars and sweeteners)
 • Convenience foods
 • Genetically modified, organic and functional foods

3 **Meal planning**
 • Balanced diets
 • Nutritional needs of different groups of people

4 **Food preparation and cooking**
 • Why food is cooked
 • Different methods of cooking
 • Effects of cooking on nutrients
 • Changes that take place when food is cooked
 • Effects of acids and alkalis on foods
 • Food additives

5 **Food safety and preservation**
 • Types of food preservation
 • The causes of food spoilage
 • Principles of food hygiene and safety
 • Food poisoning

6 **Consumer education**
 • Marketing and advertising food
 • Shopping for food
 • Food labelling
 • Laws that protect the consumer

The written examination will ask you a **variety** of questions from **each** unit of learning, so you need to make sure that you have revised and learned all of the information.

GENERAL ADVICE FOR ANSWERING A WRITTEN EXAM:

Before you start writing:

1 **Read** all the instructions on the front of the exam paper.
2 **Read** the questions carefully once, twice and then again to make sure you know **what you are being asked to do.**
3 Underline or highlight **key words** to help you focus your answer.
4 Be aware of **how many marks** each question is worth, and therefore how many facts or responses you need to give.

5 Get to know the **key words** or **command words** that will be used in the exam, such as the words shown in the following table.

Key word	What it means you should do
Identify/suggest/give reasons	Write down a list
Describe	Give details about something, e.g. how something works or what it looks like
Explain	Identify a point, write down the meaning of it clearly, then follow it with reasons to show that you understand it
Analyse	Separate a topic into its various parts in order to be able to identify and explain it
Evaluate	Assess a topic and say why it is important or what you have learned from it
Discuss	Write about all aspects of a topic, including advantages and disadvantages, or arguments for and against

TYPES OF QUESTIONS

Structured questions

These types of questions usually give you a piece of information (for example a picture or diagram, a food label, a recipe), and then ask you specific questions about it. You are given spaces in which to write the answers, and the number of marks each question is worth is put at the end in brackets.

Here is an example. (Have a go at answering the questions.)

1 Look at the recipe below for a savoury cheese and bacon flan, then answer the questions.

Savoury cheese and bacon flan

Ingredients

Short crust pastry:
200g soft plain white flour
100g shortening, e.g. butter
10tsp cold water

Filling:
4 eggs
150ml whole milk
100g strong cheddar cheese, grated
75g chopped streaky bacon, fried
1 medium onion, finely chopped and fried
Ground black pepper

Oven temperature:
To blind bake the pastry case: 200°C/Gas 6
To cook the filling: 180°C/Gas 4

---

a) Identify three ways in which the recipe could be adapted to add more fibre (NSP). (3)

b) Identify three ways in which the recipe could be adapted to reduce the fat content. (3)

c) Explain why eggs are added to the savoury flan. (3)

d) Explain why the pastry is called 'short crust'.   (2)

e) Explain why the pastry case is baked blind.   (1)

f) Explain why someone with coronary heart disease would be advised
    not to eat this flan too often.   (2)

g) Describe one way in which this flan could be adapted for a vegetarian.   (1)

Advice for answering this type of question:

- The marks awarded (in brackets) give you a clue as to **how many facts** you
  need to write down.
- Make sure that you give **specific, clear answers** – not vague or general ones.
  For example, to explain why eggs are added to the flan, an answer such as
  'because they are good for you' is too vague.
- Keep **referring back** to the information you have been given in the question to
  make sure your answers are **focused** on it.
- Even if you are not sure about the answer, have a guess and write
  something down.

Data response questions

These types of questions usually give you some data, for example in a chart,
table or pie chart, then ask specific questions about it, often with some extra
questions about the subject of the data.

Here is an example.

2 In a primary school, 64 children in two classes were asked to name their
   favourite fruits.

Fruit	Number of children who chose this fruit	% of the children who chose this fruit
Apples	12	19%
Bananas	20	31%
Grapes	9	14%
Kiwi fruit	4	6%
Mangoes	3	5%
Oranges	8	12.5%
Strawberries	8	12.5%

a) What percentage (%) of the children chose apples?   (1)

b) How many children chose grapes?   (1)

c) What percentage (%) of the children chose oranges?   (1)

d) How many children chose strawberries?   (1)

e) Which fruit was the most popular?   (1)

f) Which fruit was the least popular?   (1)

g) The school will use the information to help them decide which fruits to give children for their morning break. Give two reasons why the Government is encouraging schools to provide children with fruit to eat. (2)

h) Suggest two ways of encouraging children to eat fruit. (2)

Advice for answering this type of question:

- The marks awarded (in brackets) give you a clue as to **how many facts** or **responses** you need to write down.
- Keep **referring back** to the data you have been given to make sure your answers are **focused** on it.
- Use the evidence from the data, plus your own knowledge, to support your answer.

Free response questions

These types of questions ask you to write about a specific topic, but leave it up to you to decide the structure of your answer, which should include facts, examples and opinions.

These types of questions often include the words 'explain', 'describe' or 'discuss'.

This is what they mean:

- **Explain** – identify a point, write down the meaning of it in a clear way then follow it with reasons to show that you understand it.
- **Describe** – give details about something, for example how something works or what it looks like.
- **Discuss** – write about all aspects of a topic, including advantages and disadvantages, or arguments for and against – this shows that you have thought carefully about something, have an opinion about it and are also aware of other points of view.

Here is an example of a free response question.

3 Obesity is now a major health problem in the UK.
  - Identify some of the reasons for the increase in obesity in this country.
  - Explain why being obese is unhealthy.
  - Discuss the importance of healthy eating habits in the prevention of obesity. (15 marks)

Advice for answering this type of question:

- The marks awarded (in brackets) give you a clue as to **how many facts** or **responses** you need to include in your answer. This particular question has been split into three parts, so you should answer each part equally (in this case, include five facts or responses in each part).
- Before you start writing, make a **plan** of what you want to write about, and try to keep to it – this will help you to focus your answer.
- Keep **referring back** to the question you have been given to make sure your answer is **focused** on it.
- The quality of your **written communication** in your answer will be assessed, so you must make sure that you write **clearly**, using **good English** and without repeating what you have already said.

ACTIVITY

Try these practice exam questions.

1 Look at the chart below, which lists the ingredients for three brands of sausage, then answer the questions that follow.

Brand A	Brand B	Brand C
Pork and beef (51%), cereal rusk (wheat flour, salt), salt, white pepper, preservative, colouring, flavourings, antioxidant	Pork (89%), breadcrumb (wheat flour, salt, yeast), salt, black pepper, dried onion, preservative, nutmeg, chilli powder, coriander, antioxidant	Turkey meat (60%), water, breadcrumb (wheat flour, salt, yeast), salt, black pepper, dried onion, preservative, antioxidant

   a) Which sausage contains the most meat? (1 mark)
   b) Which sausage contains the least meat? (1 mark)
   c) Which sausage contains spices (apart from pepper)? (1 mark)
   d) Which sausage contains water? (1 mark)
   e) Which sausage can be eaten by followers of Hinduism, Islam, Judaism and Rastafarianism? (1 mark)
   f) Food manufacturers try to produce foods that help consumers follow the dietary guidelines. Explain which of the sausages above would be suitable for someone trying to follow the 'eat less fat' guideline, and how they could be cooked to limit their fat content. (3 marks)

2 Convenience foods form a large part of the diet of many people in the UK.
  • Identify the types of convenience food that are available.
  • Discuss the advantages and disadvantages of using convenience foods. (12 marks)

INDEX